Pubertal Suppression in Transgender Youth

Pubertal Suppression in Transgender Youth

COURTNEY FINLAYSON, MD
Attending Physician
Divison of Endocrinology
Ann & Robert H. Lurie Children's Hospital of Chicago
Chicago, IL, United States

Assistant Professor
Department of Pediatrics
Northwestern University Feinberg School of Medicine
Chicago, IL, United States

ELSEVIER

ELSEVIER

3251 Riverport Lane
St. Louis, Missouri 63043

Content Strategist: Nancy Duffy
Content Development Manager: Christine McElvenny
Content Development Specialist: Jennifer Horigan
Publishing Services Manager: Deepthi Unni
Project Manager: Janish Ashwin Paul
Designer: Gopalakrishnan Venkatraman

Working together
to grow libraries in
developing countries

www.elsevier.com • www.bookaid.org

Printed in United States of America
Last digit is the print number: 9 8 7 6 5 4 3 2 1

List of Contributors

Jeremi M. Carswell, MD
Instructor in Medicine
Division of Endocrinology
Boston Children's Hospital
Boston, MA, United States

Diane Chen, PhD
Assistant Professor
Department of Psychiatry and Behavioral Sciences
Northwestern University Feinberg School of Medicine
Chicago, IL, United States

Assistant Professor
Department of Pediatrics
Northwestern University Feinberg School of Medicine
Chicago, IL, United States

Medical Psychologist
Department of Child & Adolescent Psychiatry
Ann & Robert H. Lurie Children's Hospital of Chicago
Chicago, IL, United States

Medical Psychologist
Division of Adolescent Medicine
Department of Pediatrics
Ann & Robert H. Lurie Children's Hospital of Chicago
Chicago, IL, United States

Erica Eugster, MD
Professor of Pediatrics
Pediatrics
Riley Hospital for Children
Indianapolis, IN, United States

Joel E. Frader, MD, MA
Professor of Pediatrics and Professor of Bioethics and
   Medical Humanities
Feinberg School of Medicine, Northwestern University

Division Head, Pediatric Palliative Care
Ann & Robert H. Lurie Children's Hospital
Chicago, IL, United States

Anisha Gohil, DO
Pediatric Endocrinology Fellow
Pediatric Endocrinology
Riley Hospital for Children
Indianapolis, IN, United States

Rebecca M. Harris, MD, PhD, MA
Pediatric Endocrinology Fellow
Division of Endocrinology
Department of Pediatrics
Boston Children's Hospital
Boston, MA, United States

Marco A. Hidalgo, PhD
Clinical Psychologist
Center for Transyouth Health and Development
Division of Adolescent and Youth Adult Medicine
Children's Hospital Los Angeles
Los Angeles, CA, United States

Assistant Professor of Clinical Pediatrics
Keck School of Medicine
University of Southern California
Los Angeles, CA, United States

Janet Y. Lee, MD, MPH
Clinical Fellow, Adult and Pediatric Endocrinology
Divisions of Endocrinology and Metabolism and
   Pediatric Endocrinology
Departments of Medicine and Pediatrics
University of California, San Francisco
San Francisco, CA, United States

Maja Marinkovic, MD
Assistant Professor of Pediatrics
Department of Pediatric Endocrinology
University of California San Diego
San Diego, CA, United States

Leena Nahata, MD
Associate Professor of Clinical Pediatrics
The Ohio State University College of Medicine
Division of Endocrinology
Nationwide Children's Hospital
Columbus, OH, United States

Center for Biobehavioral Health
The Research Institute at Nationwide Children's
    Hospital
Columbus, OH, United States

Liat Perl, MD
Clinical Fellow
Pediatric Endocrinology
Department of Pediatrics
Meir Medical Center
Kfar Saba, Israel

Stephanie A. Roberts, MD
Boston Children's Hospital
Division of Endocrine
Boston, MA, United States

Stephen M. Rosenthal, MD
Professor of Pediatrics
Division of Pediatric Endocrinology

Medical Director
Child and Adolescent Gender Center UCSF
San Francisco, CA, United States

Loren S. Schechter, MD, FACS
Visiting Clinical Professor of Surgery, The University of
    Illinois at Chicago

Director, The Center for Gender Confirmation, Weiss
    Memorial Hospital
Morton Grove, IL, United States

Rebecca B. Schechter, MD
Highland Park, IL, United States

Daniel Evan Shumer, MD, MPH
Assistant Professor
Department of Pediatrics and Communicable Diseases
University of Michigan
Ann Arbor, MI, United States

Lisa Simons, MD
Assistant Professor of Pediatrics
Division of Adolescent Medicine
Ann & Robert H. Lurie Children's Hospital of Chicago
Chicago, IL, United States

Norman Spack, MD
Associate Physician in Medicine
Emeritus, Gender Management Service

Associate Clinical Professor of Pediatrics
Harvard Medical School
Boston, MA, United States

Dennis M. Styne, MD
Yocha Dehe Chair of Pediatric Endocrinology
Pediatrics
University of California
Davis, CA, United States

Professor of Pediatrics
Pediatrics
University of California
Davis, CA, United States

Amy C. Tishelman, PhD
Departments of Endocrinology and Psychiatry
Harvard Medical School
Boston Children's Hospital
Boston, MA, United States

Anna Valentine, MD
Department of Pediatrics
The Ohio State University College of Medicine
Nationwide Children's Hospital
Columbus, OH, United States

J. Whitehead, MD
Pediatric Endocrinology Fellow
Ann & Robert H. Lurie Children's Hospital of Chicago
McGaw Medical Center of Northwestern University
Chicago, IL, United States

Contents

CHAPTER 1

History of Care of Transgender Youth

NORMAN SPACK, MD

To write about "endocrine treatment" of transgender/gender nonconforming juveniles younger than 16 years is an oxymoronic act. Prior to the past decade, gender dysphoria, like homosexuality until 1973, was considered a psychiatric disease codified in the Diagnostic and Statistical Manual of Mental Disorders. It was unthinkable that a physician would prescribe cross-sex steroids to a gender dysphoric juvenile and risk stunted growth and induce precocious puberty. The only alternative then was psychiatric referral despite the prevalence of reparative therapy and its negative attitude toward any cross-gender behavior.[1] Efficacy of reparative therapy, which has been called into question, is based on the experience of a few investigators. They posit that only a minority of dysphoric juveniles will persist as transgender at puberty, with many who desist becoming gay. These data, like most studies on prepubertal gender nonconforming youth, were skewed by the nature of the institution in which they were seen, which in the case above was a psychiatric clinic. From the perspective of transgender individuals who seek treatment for the first time as adults, the overwhelming majority recall cross-gender feelings before the age of 10 years and many before the age of 5 years.[2] However, few parents supported their child living in a cross-gender social role in public, and the price was being bullied and rejected, which contributed to self-harm and sometimes even suicide.[3]

While some care for transgender adults has historically been provided in the United States, its fragmented nature and the lack of long-term longitudinal care and insurance coverage make outcome studies challenging. The Dutch, however, have a unique ability to perform such studies: they have one treatment center in a small country with one national insurer covering 100% care, including medical, surgical, pharmaceutical, and counseling in a country that is open minded about sexuality and gender. Despite all these favorable supports, the Dutch have considered starting treatment in adults a gigantic failure. In Louis Gooren's study of 3500 patients over 20 years, the finding that 1200 had

already died was staggering. This is 51% higher than the general population, and they didn't die of hormonal causes. They succumbed to "psychosocial deaths": suicide, substance abuse, alcoholism, homelessness, underemployment, and homicide.[4,5]

Faced with these terrible outcomes for so many transgender adults, Gooren and his associates at the VU University Medical Center Amsterdam reasoned that a totally different paradigm was necessary, one that would spare carefully screened transgender adolescents the indignity of going through their genetic puberty and live as adults with a body that would not match their affirmed gender identity. They reasoned that merely starting cross-gender steroids early in puberty would have inherent difficulties. Growth would likely be stunted and the steroids would have irreversible side effects, such as infertility, and that it would be too difficult for a 10- to 12-year-old girl or a 12- to 14-year-old boy to make a knowledgeable mature judgment about these effects. The logical alternative was pubertal blockade, as had been used for decades for children with idiopathic central precocious puberty (CPP). Before the advent of GnRH analogues (GnRHa), before 1990, the treatment was 40–60 mg high-dose progesterone daily to suppress the hypothalamic-pituitary-gonadal axis. This regimen is far from perfect, with a Cushingoid appearance due to the high-dose progesterone binding to the cortisol receptor. Thus, stress dosing for illness could be necessary, and the skeletal bone age was often inadequately suppressed, limiting height potential (personal communication, John F. Crigler, Jr., MD).

The alternative treatment for CPP was begun by a collaboration between the pediatric endocrine departments of the Boston Children's Hospital and Massachusetts General Hospitals. They used GnRHa which were successful and became the standard of care.[6] The patients stopped the GnRHa at an appropriate pubertal age, went on to fully experience full pubertal development, menstruate, ovulate, and give birth. The initial cohort has been followed for 30 years.

In a seminal moment, the Amsterdam group tried GnRHa in a few transgender early adolescents (Tanner 2) on the assumption that their puberty was acting as if it were precocious and noxious. When they later added cross-sex steroids, around the age of 15 years, while the endogenous hormones were still suppressed, the physical and psychological effects were remarkably positive.[4] Their first paper outlining their treatment evaluation and protocol for patients younger than 18 years was published in the *European Journal of Endocrinology* in 2006.[7] Inclusion of GnRHa into the therapeutic "mix" over a 22-year period was published by the same authors in 2011.[8] They also reported no net loss of bone density in patients treated with GnRH after the addition of sex hormones. This was highly significant because suppressing puberty is known to reduce bone mass acquisition. Previous data, from the younger CPP patients who took GnRH for twice as long as the transgender patients, were skewed by the fact that CPP is associated with advanced bone age and bone mineral density at the time of diagnosis, and the transgender patients are not advanced in either. Although bone mass acquisition in transgender patients continues at a prepubertal rate while only on GnRH, after 2 years of added treatment with cross-sex steroids, they normalized for age and affirmed sex. However, a more recent Dutch study suggested that bone mineral density might be compromised.[9] Conceivably, the Dutch protocol which raises cross-sex steroid dose relatively slowly could be responsible, and this is a fertile area for future investigation.

In evaluation of psychosocial functioning, virtually all programs that treat using pubertal suppression have noted a marked reduction in self-harm compared to the pretreatment era. Equally important, is the remarkable outcome in psychosocial well-being for patients treated with all components of the Dutch protocol: GnRHa treatment in early puberty, gender-affirming hormones added around the age of 15 years, and all surgeries completed at the age of 18 years.[8] When individuals were studied again at the age of 20–22 years, living in the complete social role of their affirmed gender, their psychosocial well-being not only compared favorably with age-matched nontransgender Dutch peers but was also often better.[10]

Awakening the American pediatric endocrine audience to their potentially pivotal role in the care of transgender youth was no easy matter. With its designation as a psychiatric disease, many endocrine division and pediatric department leaders would have preferred that these patients remain in the psychiatric clinics. Multidisciplinary care was expensive and the probability of funding for clinical care in a medical clinic for a psychiatric disorder was questionable. Furthermore, insurance coverage for GnRHa, that cost hundreds to thousands of dollars, was invariably not covered. In the late 1990s, two conferences were held for combined European and American physicians and mental health professionals interested in becoming involved with transgender youth. At the first, in London, the Dutch team presented their plan for what became known as the "Dutch Protocol" of pubertal suppression. Shortly after, at a working group conference at VU University Medical Center Amsterdam (VUMC), Peggy Cohen-Kettenis offered to share her psychological testing materials to confirm severe gender dysphoria with the then Boston Children's Hospital psychologist Laura Edwards-Leeper, PhD. In 1998, Henriette Delemarre, MD, from VUMC presented her preliminary findings on the Dutch cohort of pubertally suppressed adolescents at an endocrine division conference at the Boston Children's Hospital and gave special attention to their preliminary studies, showing that 2 years of cross-sex hormones protected against diminished bone mineral density.

Also in 1998, this author began to bring older teens on cross-sex hormones into the Endocrine Teaching Clinic, inspiring several of the Boston Children's Hospital's endocrine fellows and some rotating internal medicine fellows to get involved. Within a decade, many of these physicians would have transgender patients of their own. In the final analysis, interacting with transgender patients and their parents convinced other physicians, mental health staff, nurses, and administrators that transgender adolescents were not mentally ill, yet were in profound danger of suicide and bullying. The patient numbers were not large enough to guarantee that they would ever knowingly see a transgender patient. Yet, many departments heard about the number of patients we were seeing and wanted to be better informed. A decision was made to let the patients do the talking, and indeed, they captured the hearts and minds of the hospital community. The hospital administration was so proud of being the first such clinic in North America that a semiannual glossy magazine sent out by the development office featured the clinic we named "GeMS," the Gender Management Service.

By 2005, the Boston clinic had an endocrinologist, a psychologist skilled in testing, and a social worker and was ready to open the doors to new patients who were gender dysphoric and between Tanner 2 and 18 years of age. To make full use of the clinic space and broaden the range of patients to be seen, half the patients were not transgender but had disorders of sex development and were cared for collaboratively by urologists and endocrinologists. Regrettably, the clinic was not yet able to provide counseling and support groups for younger or prepubertal children, and for the immediate high demand for the new services provided.

The clinic was a favorite for observation by medical students and residents from a variety of disciplines. Since the clinic session lasted a whole day, cases of the day were discussed with the entire team during a lunch conference including the medical "visitors." Several of the attendees at the clinic, like Stanley Vance, MD, have made their marks as leaders of new programs for transgender adolescents around the continent. Vance began coming to our clinic as a first-year Harvard Medical student and is now on the adolescent medicine staff of the University of California, San Francisco (UCSF), and a key figure in that Center's gender team. He spent a year with the Amsterdam group on a Fulbright grant while in medical school and coauthored papers with us.

Our 2012 *Pediatrics* publication described our first 100 consecutive patients.[2] Noteworthy findings were the advanced age and degree of pubertal advancement in genotypic females, averaging 15 years of age. Most patients described feelings of being in the wrong body as early as the age of 5 years. Forty-four percent had significant psychiatric histories, 20% reported self-mutilation and 9% had made suicide attempts. For the past 5 years, the GeMS program has sponsored one weekend day annually for each of the three groups: families, health professionals, and school personnel. Since 2015, with additional staff, prepubertal children are being seen. Perhaps the most significant impact of the GeMS clinic is the encouragement provided to other clinicians across the nation who wished to create a similar clinic of their own. In 2007, GeMS was the sole clinic in any pediatric academic center on the continent. A decade later, there are approximately 60 programs, and the GeMS provided advice to most of them.

In 2008 a task force led by Wylie Hembree, MD, was appointed by the President of the Endocrine Society to compose "Guidelines for Treatment of Transgender Adults and Adolescents." For adolescents, the Guidelines endorsed the Dutch protocol of pubertal suppression using GnRHa. The document was ratified by the Society membership and published in its main clinical journal, *The Journal of Clinical Endocrinology and Metabolism*, in 2009 and as a separate monograph.[11] This was the first time that a major international journal had devoted such concern for the medical well-being of the transgender adolescent population, and it

provided professional support at the highest level for physicians working in academic medical centers. Now, there are papers and symposia at every Endocrine Society annual meeting and in other society meetings such as the Society for Adolescent Health and Medicine, the American College Health Association, and the Pediatric Endocrine Society as well as others. Colleges and universities, especially those that were self-insured, began to extend specific medical care and, in some cases, full surgical benefits to transgender students. Several prominent women's colleges that had already accepted applicants who had transitioned to their affirmed female gender also allowed enrolled students who were accepted as women but transitioned to men once they had matriculated.

In 2010 Nick Teich established Camp Aranu'tiq as a week-long summer overnight camp in a rented space in southern New England, serving 40 campers. It was the first-ever summer camp established for transgender and gender-variant/gender-nonconforming youth. Camp and travel costs were free for all those who needed it and campers came from as far as Hawaii. Many of the staff were transgender or gender-variant. For the first time in this "regular" camp, transgender campers met other individuals like themselves, developing firm friendships which lasted well beyond the camp week via social media. After the camp, 82% of campers said they felt more confident in themselves than before attending Aranu'tiq. In 2014, Teich and his board purchased a 116-acre New Hampshire property and added 4 weeks of camping to serve 500 campers and off-season family weekends in a heated main building.

In 2014, this author was asked to do an 18-minute TedTalk, "How I help transgender teens be who they want to be." By 2017, it had 2 million views and had become a teaching instrument in universities and high schools.

In 2015, the National Institutes of Health announced a multimillion dollar grant for the first multicenter longitudinal 4-year study of adolescents to study the long-term impact of early medical care for transgender youth. Awardees were the Ann & Robert H. Lurie Children's Hospital of Chicago, UCSF, Children's Hospital of Los Angeles, and CHB. Also in 2015, Ximena Lopez, MD, and Jerry Olshan, MD, with the assistance of Steve Rosenthal, MD, President of the Pediatric Endocrine Society, obtained "Special Interest Group" status for attendees at the Society meetings. This guaranteed that time and space will always be available for those who wish to meet about transgender care.

By 2017, many directors of gender clinics noticed a change in the population of new patients coming through their front doors. Far more claimed to be "gender fluid" or "gender queer" and showed little interest in evaluation. Rather, parents of the youth seeking help raising an adolescent who does not identify in a binary fashion. This patient group presents new challenges for providers as well, in tailoring potential interventions to the individual's desires.

All the above success belies the reality that improvement in care is not evenly distributed to transgender youth across the United States. Access to care and insurance coverage are limited by insufficient training and knowledge which are sometimes fueled by cultural and religious beliefs and sometimes coalesce into political prejudices. This varies by state and mapping clinics by states looks like the red and blue national election map. The operating clinics are overly distributed on the more liberal coasts, and large centers in the center and south are left without services. But, worst of all, we are experiencing direct antipathy and discrimination at the highest level of our government, manifest in restrictions of restroom rights and attempts to deny service in our military to transgender people.

We have so far to go, and taking care of transgender people requires more than prescriptions. It requires advocacy and a commitment to educating medical students, trainees, and our peers.

DEDICATION
Dedicated to the memory of Henriette Delemarre, MD, who taught us by example in pure collaboration.

REFERENCES

1. Zucker KJ. On the "natural history" of gender identity disorder in children. *J Am Acad Child Adolesc Psychiatry*. 2008;47(12):1361–1363. https://doi.org/10.1097/CHI.0b013e31818960cf.
2. Spack NP, Edwards-Leeper L, Feldman HA, et al. Children and adolescents with gender identity disorder referred to a pediatric medical center. *Pediatrics*. 2012;129(3):418–425. https://doi.org/10.1542/peds.2011-0907.
3. Dhejne C, Lichtenstein P, Boman M, Johansson AL, Langstrom N, Landen M. Long-term follow-up of transsexual persons undergoing sex reassignment surgery: cohort study in Sweden. *PLoS One*. 2011;6(2):e16885. https://doi.org/10.1371/journal.pone.0016885.
4. Asscheman H, Giltay EJ, Megens JA, de Ronde WP, van Trotsenburg MA, Gooren LJ. A long-term follow-up study of mortality in transsexuals receiving treatment with cross-sex hormones. *Eur J Endocrinol*. 2011;164(4):635–642. https://doi.org/10.1530/EJE-10-1038.
5. Grossman AH, D'Augelli AR. Transgender youth and life-threatening behaviors. *Suicide Life Threat Behav*. 2007;37(5):527–537. https://doi.org/10.1521/suli.2007.37.5.527.
6. Boepple PA, Mansfield MJ, Wierman ME, et al. Use of a potent, long acting agonist of gonadotropin-releasing hormone in the treatment of precocious puberty. *Endocr Rev*. 1986;7(1):24–33. https://doi.org/10.1210/edrv-7-1-24.
7. Delemarre-van de Waal H, Cohen-Kettenis P. Clinical management of gender identity disorder in adolescents: a protocol on psychological and paediatric endocrinology aspects. *Eur J Endocrinol*. 2006;155:S131–S137.
8. Kreukels BP, Cohen-Kettenis PT. Puberty suppression in gender identity disorder: the Amsterdam experience. *Nat Rev Endocrinol*. 2011;7(8):466–472. https://doi.org/10.1038/nrendo.2011.78.
9. Klink D, Caris M, Heijboer A, van Trotsenburg M, Rotteveel J. Bone mass in young adulthood following gonadotropin-releasing hormone analog treatment and cross-sex hormone treatment in adolescents with gender dysphoria. *J Clin Endocrinol Metab*. 2015;100(2):E270–E275. https://doi.org/10.1210/jc.2014-2439.
10. de Vries AL, McGuire JK, Steensma TD, Wagenaar EC, Doreleijers TA, Cohen-Kettenis PT. Young adult psychological outcome after puberty suppression and gender reassignment. *Pediatrics*. 2014;134(4):696–704. https://doi.org/10.1542/peds.2013-2958.
11. Hembree WC, Cohen-Kettenis P, Delemarre-van de Waal HA, et al. Endocrine treatment of transsexual persons: an Endocrine Society clinical practice guideline. *J Clin Endocrinol Metab*. 2009;94(9):3132–3154. https://doi.org/10.1210/jc.2009-0345.

CHAPTER 2

Models of Care and Current Guidelines for Care of Transgender Individuals

J. WHITEHEAD, MD • LISA SIMONS, MD

As general awareness about gender diversity has increased over the past decade, more transgender and gender-diverse (TGD) youth and their families are seeking gender-related education, support, and medical and mental healthcare services. The terms "transgender" and "gender-diverse" describe youth whose gender identity, gender expression, and/or behaviors do not align with culturally defined norms for their birth-assigned sex.[1] In response to the growing need to support these youth, the number of pediatric clinics providing specialized care to TGD youth has steadily increased across the United States in recent years. Though we are far from a universal consensus, the gender-affirming approach is increasingly embraced as the optimal approach to management of *gender dysphoria*, a term referring to the emotional distress that may arise due to incongruence between an individual's birth-assigned sex and gender identity.[2,3] In addition, it is widely agreed upon that comprehensive care for TGD youth is best delivered by a multidisciplinary team that includes medical and mental healthcare clinicians who have experience working with children and adolescents.[4,5] The authors of this section join with many specialized pediatric gender clinics, health organizations, and medical societies across the United States who embrace a "gender-affirming" approach to care. In this chapter, we define gender-affirming care, discuss components of a comprehensive multidisciplinary program model, and review clinical practice guidelines (CPG) for treating gender dysphoria in adolescence.

GENDER-AFFIRMING CARE

The gender-affirming approach acknowledges a wide spectrum of gender identities and expressions beyond the gender binary (a system which recognizes only two genders—male and female). The gender-affirming approach also recognizes that gender expression and

identity may be fluid and change over time within an individual.[6] Although gender nonconforming identities and expressions may transgress cultural norms, the gender-affirming model views the gender spectrum as part of the human experience and does not regard gender diversity as pathologic.[6] These foundational tenets of the gender-affirming model of care inform every interaction with transgender youth.

"Gender affirmation" refers broadly to any interaction that recognizes, validates, and supports a person's experienced gender identity and gender expression. For example, using a person's preferred name and gender pronouns is a form of gender affirmation. Allowing youth the opportunity to play on the sports team of their experienced gender and use locker rooms or restrooms consistent with their experienced gender are other examples of gender affirmation. Gender-affirming care neither views gender nonconformity as a mental illness nor presumes the trajectory of any gender nonconforming youth's gender identity. Rather, gender-affirming care posits that all youth deserve a safe space for active gender exploration.[6]

Unlike a corrective approach, which redirects gender nonconforming behaviors or expressions with the goal of reducing them and ultimately aligning gender behavior and identity with one's birth-assigned sex, the gender-affirming approach promotes gender exploration and supports youth living in the way that is most comfortable for them.[6] TGD people represent a heterogeneous group of people with different goals and desires for themselves. The gender-affirming approach recognizes that not all TGD people experience gender dysphoria. For those who do, *transitioning*, the process by which one begins to live in their affirmed gender role, may alleviate distress and improve well-being.[7–9] Thus, the gender-affirming model recognizes the need for an individualized approach to care, and all interventions (social, medical, and surgical) are implemented with the goal of reducing an individual's gender dysphoria.[2] Gender-affirming clinicians often educate patients with gender dysphoria and their families about options for transitioning and support them as they make decisions about their future.

Long-term prospective research on the impact of gender-affirming care for TGD youth is needed to better inform clinical practice. To date, several studies examining the impact of gender-affirming care for gender dysphoria have demonstrated associations with positive outcomes. For example, one study of socially transitioned prepubertal transgender children showed that they did not have higher depression scores and had only marginally higher anxiety scores than age-matched cisgender children.[9] A Canadian study of transgender youth showed that those who reported strong parental support also reported higher self-esteem and more positive mental health.[10] Gender-affirming treatment for gender dysphoria has also been associated with decreased rates of adverse negative psychosocial outcomes such as depression, suicidality, and homelessness.[6] While research regarding long-term clinical outcomes of those receiving gender-affirming care is lacking, these early studies reflect the experience of gender-affirming specialists, who observe that youth who are accepted and supported by family and community and who are given the opportunity to live as they feel most comfortable are less likely to experience distress.

MULTIDISCIPLINARY CARE

The multidisciplinary care model is widely used for chronic pediatric conditions.[11] Multidisciplinary clinics increase communication between providers to deliver more comprehensive, efficient, and organized care. For patients seeing multiple providers, this model may also reduce the burdens associated with travel costs and time off from work and/or school.[11]

The archetype of a multidisciplinary pediatric gender program first opened its doors in 1987 at the VU University Medical Center in Amsterdam, Netherlands, and is now called the Center of Expertise on Gender Dysphoria.[12] In the United States, the first multidisciplinary gender clinics for TGD youth emerged in the mid- to late-2000s, and the number of clinics has steadily increased over the past decade.[13] Multidisciplinary clinics not only provide medical and mental healthcare but may also offer nonclinical services, including, but not limited to, peer and parent support groups, referrals for legal assistance, and school-related advocacy.[1] These ancillary services, described in greater detail in subsequent sections, often make powerful differences in youths' daily lives.

PRACTICE GUIDELINES

Currently, two publications offer recommendations to clinicians on the provision of care to TGD people, each with sections specifically focused on care for children and adolescents. Both publications are based on the best available research and expert consensus. In 1979, the World Professional Association for Transgender Health (WPATH) published its first Standards of Care (SOC) which is currently in its seventh version.[5] The WPATH SOC aim to be comprehensive in their discussion of gender-affirming treatment for transgender and gender-nonconforming people and include recommendations for various health professionals working with this population. The WPATH SOC categorize medical treatment for gender dysphoria into fully reversible, partially reversible, or irreversible interventions and also outline the roles of mental health professionals. In September 2017, the Endocrine Society published *Endocrine Treatment of Gender Dysphoric/Gender Incongruent Persons*, an update to their 2009 CPG.[4,14] The Endocrine Society Clinical Practice Guideline (CPG), which focus primarily on medical treatment of individuals experiencing gender dysphoria, distinguish evidence-based recommendations from value judgments or practice preferences of experts in the field.

Both sets of guidelines are meant to serve as flexible frameworks for providers, and clinicians are encouraged to apply the guidelines while simultaneously taking into account individual considerations and the sociocultural context. The guidelines have undergone and will continue to undergo revisions as both the scientific basis of recommendations and the cultural landscape in which care is provided continue to evolve. The remainder of this chapter will discuss the provision of gender-affirming care for transgender youth in a multidisciplinary setting, referring to these guidelines as applicable to the current practice landscape.

MENTAL HEALTHCARE

Identifying as transgender or expressing gender identity in ways that do not conform to cultural expectations is not "wrong" or pathologic. While gender incongruence or nonconformity alone should never be considered a form of mental illness, many (but not all) TGD youth do experience psychosocial stressors and mental health issues, which are believed to be related in great part to society's treatment of TGD people. For example, transgender youth may suffer rejection due to their gender identity or expression on an interpersonal level (e.g., family members, peers), a community level (e.g., school, spiritual/faith group), and a systemic level (e.g., discriminatory government policies). In addition, TGD youth commonly face verbal harassment, physical assault, and bullying both in person and online.[15,16] Lack of financial support and inadequate housing are other common psychosocial challenges for TGD youth.[15,16] Several studies have reported high rates of mental health concerns in TGD youth seeking care, most frequently depression and anxiety.[17,18] Mental health concerns and needs of TGD adolescents vary, and treatment should be individualized to each patient's unique needs.

Thus, mental health clinicians are essential members of the multidisciplinary care model for transgender youth. The roles of mental health professionals working with children and adolescents with gender dysphoria as outlined in the WPATH SOC are (1) assessment of gender dysphoria, (2) provision of family counseling and supportive psychotherapy to assist with exploring gender identity, (3) assessment and treatment of coexisting mental health concerns, (4) referral to medical providers for consideration of transition services, (5) education and advocacy on behalf of children with gender dysphoria, and (6) referral for peer and parent support groups.[5] For TGD youth who are not gender dysphoric, providing education and support for patients and families is the primary role, and referral to medical providers for physical transitioning is not indicated.

Families present to gender clinics for various reasons and with varying amounts of knowledge or familiarity with phenomenology related to gender. Therapists frequently provide psychoeducation about gender development, gender expression and identity, and gender dysphoria. Family-based therapy may be useful when family members struggle to understand or accept a youth's gender identity or expression or do not know how to respond to a youth's gender nonconformity. Youth who are questioning their gender identity may benefit from individual therapy with a mental health clinician focused on gender exploration.

Mental health professionals routinely assess for the presence of gender dysphoria and educate patients and families about possible interventions to reduce gender dysphoria. The Diagnostic and Statistical Manual of Mental Disorders (DSM) provides specific criteria for the diagnosis of gender dysphoria in children and adolescents,[2] and mental health providers should be competent in using the DSM.

Families may present to a multidisciplinary gender clinic to learn more about social transitioning. There is no one "right way" or "right time" for youth to socially transition. The decision to socially transition is a personal one made by each patient and family, and an individualized plan for transitioning should aim to lessen discomfort while taking into account factors such as patient preferences and personal safety. Patients may choose to make any of a number of reversible changes, including changing their name, preferred gender pronouns, or elements of their gender expression or presentation such as clothing or haircut. Increasingly, children initially presenting to multidisciplinary gender clinics for care have already socially transitioned,[4] and the limited evidence available to date has demonstrated positive mental health outcomes for early social transition.[9] Mental health clinicians may support patients undergoing social transition and help families navigate common issues such as how to disclose to school and family members.

For gender dysphoric youth who have entered puberty and who meet eligibility criteria, gender-affirming medical treatment may be administered with the goal of alleviating gender dysphoria. (For pre-pubertal TGD youth, medical treatment is not indicated.[4]) The Endocrine Society CPG recommend that "all clinicians referring youth for services should be knowledgeable about the diagnostic criteria for gender-affirming treatment, have sufficient training and experience in assessing psychopathology, and be willing to participate in the ongoing care throughout the transition."[4] Mental health clinicians play a role in educating patients about medical interventions and in assessing readiness to begin treatment.[4,5] In a readiness assessment, the mental health provider: (1) documents the diagnosis of gender dysphoria, (2) confirms that any mental health conditions or psychosocial concerns that might interfere with treatment have been reasonably addressed and do not compromise the patient's ability to make an informed decision, and (3) evaluates the patient's capacity to provide informed consent or assent. In order to do so, providers must assess the patient's knowledge of the desired intervention (including side effects and known and unknown risks, benefits, and alternatives) and confirm that the patient has reasonable expectations of the desired treatment.

While ongoing psychotherapy is not mandated for youth receiving medical treatment for gender dysphoria, it is strongly recommended that mental healthcare be available to support youth before, during, and after transitioning.[4] TGD may benefit from therapy focused on developing coping skills to counteract marginalization or stigma experienced due to gender nonconformity.[1] Youth with concomitant mental health issues may benefit from engaging in ongoing mental health treatment related to their specific mental health conditions. As for all youth regardless of their gender identity, psychiatric services may be indicated for conditions such as depression, anxiety, posttraumatic stress disorder, or attention-deficit/hyperactivity disorder. It can be exceptionally challenging for transgender youth to work with providers who are not gender-affirming since rapport between patient and provider is vital to treatment success. Thus, identifying gender-affirming and culturally sensitive psychologic and psychiatric providers, either within or outside of the multidisciplinary team, is crucial to optimizing management of these conditions.

MEDICAL CARE

Upon presentation to a gender clinic, clinicians collect gender development history and assess for the presence of gender dysphoria. In some multidisciplinary clinics, mental health providers and medical staff meet with families and collect this information together.[1] Treatment is individualized and targeted at reducing distress, when present. For some youth, gender-affirming psychotherapy or social interventions may be sufficient to reduce gender dysphoria, but for others, the experience of an undesired puberty and the resulting incongruence between one's experienced gender identity and physical appearance can be unbearable. Early medical intervention to reduce gender dysphoria after puberty has begun may prevent psychological harm.[4]

Gender-affirming medical interventions include pubertal suppression with gonadotropin-releasing hormone agonists (GnRHa) and gender-affirming hormones (estrogen or testosterone). Pubertal suppression is a reversible intervention that may be indicated for youth whose long-lasting gender dysphoria intensifies with puberty or for youth who are in the process of exploring their gender identity and who are distressed by puberty.[4,5] Suppression of endogenous sex hormones by GnRHa pauses puberty and, when administered early, prevents the development of undesired and sometimes irreversible physical changes. Pubertal suppression provides an opportunity for youth to explore their gender or to continue living in their affirmed gender without the distress associated with ongoing pubertal development before they are ready to make decisions about partially irreversible treatments (such as estrogen or testosterone). For older adolescents who meet the eligibility criteria, gender-affirming hormones are used to reduce endogenous sex hormones and replace them with those that more accurately match one's affirmed gender, thereby inducing secondary sexual characteristics that are more aligned with one's gender identity and desired gender expression.

Current practice guidelines are based on the best available research and also recognize expert opinion in areas where research is insufficient. Both the Endocrine Society CPG and WPATH SOC describe the rationale for use of gender-affirming medical interventions and specify the eligibility criteria to be met prior to initiating treatment.[4,5] The Endocrine Society CPG offer clinicians guidance for management, including timing of initiation of medical intervention, baseline bloodwork and imaging, as well as protocols for medication dosing and monitoring.[4]

Medical providers with different specialties or training may participate in the multidisciplinary care of TGD youth, including pediatric endocrinologists, general pediatricians, adolescent medicine specialists, and nurse practitioners or other mid-level providers. All clinicians should have a specific interest and expertise in treating gender dysphoria and experience working with children and adolescents.

Endocrinologists play an important role in the management of pubertal suppression and gender-affirming hormones, monitoring Tanner stage, gonadotropin and sex steroid levels, metabolic parameters, bone density, and growth rate. Adolescent medicine specialists may also have experience managing medical treatment of gender dysphoria. In addition, they offer knowledge of sexual and reproductive health, adolescent development, symptomatology of mood disorders, and screening for high-risk behaviors, which are essential health services. All medical providers involved in the management of gender dysphoria should provide accurate and comprehensive counseling regarding the desired medical treatment's potential benefits, known and unknown risks, side effects, and alternatives. It is helpful to assess patients' understanding and expectations of medications. Counseling should review the treatment's anticipated effects in detail, including the reversibility of each effect, the anticipated timeline along which effects will occur, and how the intervention might impact future considerations such as gender-affirming surgical treatment or fertility. CPG highlight the responsibility that providers have to counsel patients about options for fertility preservation prior to initiating treatment.[4,5] Patients and families who are interested in pursuing fertility preservation or learning more about fertility preservation options should be referred to reproductive endocrinologists or urologists for consultation.

Gender-affirming surgeries may be necessary to alleviate gender dysphoria for some TGD individuals; therefore, surgeons are valued members of a multidisciplinary care team. Surgical procedures address an individual's unique experience of dysphoria with the goal of reducing discomfort and allowing the patient to more easily integrate into society in their affirmed gender role. Desired surgeries may include various genital surgeries, breast augmentation, mastectomy, facial feminization surgeries, chondrolaryngoplasty, and vocal cord surgeries. Plastic surgeons, otolaryngologists, urologists, and gynecologists are among the providers who may be trained in these procedures. Current guidelines recommend that patients desiring surgery reach a minimum age of 18 years or the legal age of majority in their country due to the irreversibility of the procedures.[4,5] The sole area of greater flexibility is mastectomy, for which guidelines acknowledge that there is insufficient evidence to recommend an age requirement and suggest clinicians determine appropriate timing for surgical referral.[5,14] Per practice guidelines, at least one readiness assessment conducted by a mental health provider is required prior to surgery and is analogous to the process described previously for initiating medical treatment.

Primary care providers (PCPs) can play a critical role in ensuring that TGD youth receive appropriate care. PCPs conduct age-appropriate screening for depression and anxiety, self-harm, disordered eating, family conflict, and substance use. They provide family planning and contraception services, complete organ-specific screening, and encourage routine wellness such as counseling on nutrition and physical activity. Often, PCPs have trusted relationships with families and may be a parent's first source of guidance regarding their child's gender nonconformity. Pediatricians may identify youth in their practice who are struggling with gender and provide reassurance, education, support, and referrals for gender-affirming medical or mental healthcare.[19] When families are unable to access care at a multidisciplinary gender clinic, some PCPs, depending on their experience and comfort level working with TGD youth, may be willing to co-manage medical treatment for gender dysphoria in consultation with pediatric endocrinologists or other specialists. Other PCPs may provide medical services such as menstrual suppression to adolescents with gender dysphoria associated with menses. Pediatricians may facilitate necessary referrals and coordinate clinical and laboratory monitoring of youth receiving hormonal treatment at specialized gender clinics.

All clinicians caring for TGD youth should be familiar with nonhormonal and nonsurgical strategies used by some individuals to reduce not only gender dysphoria but also social anxiety related to "passing" and risk of harassment and violence that can result from being perceived as transgender or gender nonconforming. For those who have undergone an estrogen-mediated puberty, chest binders may reduce the appearance of breast tissue. Chest binding may be associated with pain, skin irritation, and restriction of movement and lung expansion[20]; therefore, providing patients with guidance regarding safe binding strategies is critical. Some community programs and clinics have organized binder exchanges, as purchasing binders can be cost-prohibitive for youth. For patients who have undergone a testosterone-mediated puberty, facial hair may cause distress and clinicians may provide referrals for hair removal services such as laser treatment or electrolysis. Transgender women may also seek information on safe ways to "tuck" their genitals in order to conceal their appearance. It is important to be aware that some materials used for tucking can cause skin irritation. Individuals of all gender identities may benefit from vocal training services to learn strategies to self-modulate their voice without incurring vocal damage.[5]

ADJUNCTIVE SERVICES

TGD and their families may benefit from a number of nonclinical services that support patient well-being. Services continue to evolve in multidisciplinary gender clinics in response to identified patient/family needs. For instance, one multidisciplinary clinic has described their experience in developing popular services such as a vocal therapy group led by a speech therapist and a wellness group led by a personal trainer focused on exercise training and nutritional counseling.[1]

While the number of gender-diverse children being referred for gender-affirming medical care is increasing, many youth and their caregivers feel isolated. Youth and parent/caregiver support groups provide a space for people to share experiences and strategies navigating specific issues and to develop a community of support. Some specialized gender programs have formed their own support groups for children, adolescents, young adults, siblings, and parents/caregivers, while other programs connect interested families with local community-based groups. Either approach can achieve the same goal of fostering a support network for patients and families who might otherwise feel isolated.[1]

For gender-diverse youth, school settings are often stressful and sometimes dangerous, particularly when students lack support or suffer discrimination and harassment by school administrators, teachers, and peers.[1,21] For example, in one large survey, 75% of transgender students reported feeling unsafe at school because of their gender expression, and 12% had experienced harassment or assault based on their gender expression.[21] Laws protecting students from discrimination based on gender and/or sexuality vary from state to state. Multidisciplinary programs serving youth should consider offering outreach and education to school and district personnel, who are often inadequately trained to create gender-inclusive educational settings or respond to student- or parent-led discriminatory efforts.[1] Professional development trainings can be targeted to various school personnel on topics such as respecting a student's preferred name and gender pronouns, navigating access to shared spaces (bathrooms, locker rooms), and facilitating participation in sports, which often strictly adhere to the gender binary. Clinical or nonclinical providers can play an important role by collaborating directly with school administrators, teachers, and coaches. Alternatively, gender clinics may connect families to existing local or national resources, such as nonprofit organizations that offer advocacy services for gender-diverse youth in schools and other settings. Advocacy also ideally extends to other places where youth may spend significant time—including but not limited to community-mentoring programs, foster care systems, the juvenile justice system, and homeless shelters.[22]

The WPATH SOC highlight the importance of legal knowledge in the care of transgender people and emphasize that one role of a provider is to be aware of the public policies that impact their patients' lives.[4,5] Legal consultation can be beneficial for assistance in appealing for insurance denial of gender-related healthcare, for support navigating the process of legal name and/or gender marker change, and for aid in combating discrimination. Gender clinics should be aware of the available resources for families and, whenever able, provide referrals to a network of legal support professionals in the community. In addition, depending on local legislation, medical or mental health providers are commonly asked to provide documentation in support of legal name or gender marker changes. Documentation change may also require costly processing fees,

and providers should be knowledgeable about available resources to offset the financial burden of these legal processes.

Finally, whenever possible, clinical and nonclinical staff should engage in capacity building and advocacy, on an individual or broader level. For example, mental health or medical providers with gender-related expertise can offer consultation to a patients' primary therapist or pediatrician when families are unable to access treatment in a multidisciplinary clinic or when primary providers are seeking more education.[1] Clinical and nonclinical staff may supervise trainees or conduct community training on topics relevant to their area of expertise such as pediatric gender diversity, the multidisciplinary approach to care for gender dysphoria, and cultural competency in health, school, and legal settings.[1]

BARRIERS TO CARE

Unfortunately, while transgender people continue to suffer significant health disparities, limited research has focused on the health system's capacity to address this population's healthcare needs.[23] Numerous barriers, both within and outside of the healthcare system, have been described.[23,24] Overwhelmingly, the most frequently cited barrier is a lack of access to healthcare services due to healthcare providers' lack of knowledge about gender-affirming care. In one survey of transgender adults, half of the respondents reported having to educate their medical provider about transition-related care, and over one-quarter described previously experiencing harassment in medical settings.[25] Other cited barriers include cost of care, lack of insurance coverage, inadequate transportation or long travel times to specialized clinics, and previous negative healthcare experiences.[23,24]

Electronic medical records (EMRs) pose challenges to transgender people and their care providers. For many transgender patients, sex assigned at birth, gender identity (including identities outside the binary), and the gender marker on their legal documents do not all align. Current EMR systems vary in their flexibility and ability to capture information such as preferred name and pronouns, legal name, gender identity, birth-assigned sex, and legal sex. EMR systems are hampered in that they must contain identifying and demographic information which matches the patient's insurance records for billing purposes. EMR systems must document medical history in order to provide appropriate care to the patient, while at the same time maintaining the patient's privacy.

Inadequate nuance within the EMR is further complicated by the health insurance system. In the United States, which does not offer universal healthcare, insurance coverage of gender-affirming medical care can vary widely by insurance policy and from state to state. In many if not most cases, prior authorizations are required for GnRHa and gender-affirming hormone treatments. In some cases, insurance companies have denied necessary sex-specific services based on the gender marker on the patient's insurance policy or medical chart. For example, some insurance companies have denied coverage for necessary screenings such as pap smears for transgender males whose gender marker in the EMR and on their insurance policy have been updated to match gender identity rather than sex assigned at birth. It can be helpful to have designated staff members available to provide guidance around issues which may arise due to legal documentation. Presently, the interaction between health insurance companies, EMRs, and care providers is a complicated matter for transgender patients, which, while evolving rapidly, remains far from standardized and fully integrated.

SUMMARY

The multidisciplinary approach to care offers comprehensive services aimed at optimizing the emotional and physical well-being of TGD youth. In areas where the multidisciplinary model of care is not accessible, partnering with community-based providers to deliver gender-affirming services is essential. Gender-affirming services are individualized and seek to support TGD exploring their gender identity and living as they feel most comfortable.

REFERENCES

1. Chen D, Hidalgo M, Leibowitz S, et al. Multidisciplinary care for gender-diverse youth: a narrative review and unique model of gender-affirming care. *Transgender Health.* 2016;1(1):117−123.
2. *Diagnostic and Statistical Manual of Mental Disorders, Version 5.* Washington, DC: American Psychiatric Association; 2013.
3. Drescher J, Byne W. Gender dysphoric/gender variant (GD/GV) children and adolescents: summarizing what we know and what we have yet to learn. *J Homosex.* 2012;59(3):501−510.
4. Hembree W, Cohen-Kettenis P, Gooren L, et al. Endocrine treatment of gender-dysphoric/gender-incongruent persons: an endocrine society clinical practice guideline. *J Clin Endocrinol Metab.* 2017;102(11):3869−3903.
5. Coleman E, Bockting W, Botzer M. Standards of care for the health of transsexual, transgender, and gender nonconforming people. *Int J Transgenderism.* 2011;13:165−232.
6. Hidalgo MA, Ehrensaft D, Tishelman AC, et al. The gender affirmative model: what we know and what we aim to learn. *Hum Dev.* 2013;56(5):285−290.
7. Durwood L, McLaughlin KA, Olson KR. Mental health and self-worth in socially transitioned transgender youth. *J Am Acad Child Adolesc Psychiatry.* 2017;56(2):116−123.e112.
8. White Hughto JM, Reisner SL. A systematic review of the effects of hormone therapy on psychological functioning and quality of life in transgender individuals. *Transgend Health.* 2016;1(1):21−31.
9. Olson KR, Durwood L, DeMeules M, McLaughlin KA. Mental health of transgender children who are supported in their identities. *Pediatrics.* 2016;137(3):e20153223.
10. Travers R, Bauer G, Pyne J, Bradley K, Gale L, Papadimitriou M. *Impacts of Strong Parental Support for Trans Youth: A Report Prepared by the Children's Aid Society of Toronto and Delisle Youth Services.* Toronto: Ontario; 2012.
11. Grosse S, Schechter M, Kulkarni R, Lloyd-Puryear M, Strickland B, Trevathan E. Models of comprehensive multidisciplinary care for individuals in the United States with genetic disorders. *Pediatrics.* 2009;123:407−412.
12. de Vries AL, Cohen-Kettenis PT. Clinical management of gender dysphoria in children and adolescents: the Dutch approach. *J Homosex.* 2012;59(3):301−320.
13. Sherer I, Rosenthal S, Ehrensaft D, Baum J. Child and adolescent gender center: a multidisciplinary collaboration to improve the lives of gender nonconforming children and teens. *Pediatr Rev.* 2012;33(6):273−275.
14. Hembree WC, Cohen-Kettenis P, Delemarre-van de Waal HA, et al. Endocrine treatment of transsexual persons: an endocrine society clinical practice guideline. *J Clin Endocrinol Metab.* 2009;94(9):3132−3154.
15. Grossman AH, D'Augelli AR. Transgender youth: invisible and vulnerable. *J Homosex.* 2006;51(1):111−128.
16. *American Psychological Association Task Force on Gender Identity and Gender Variance. Report of the APA Task Force on Gender Identity and Gender Variance.* Washington: DC; 2009.
17. Spack NP, Edwards-Leeper L, Feldman HA, et al. Children and adolescents with gender identity disorder referred to a pediatric medical center. *Pediatrics.* 2012;129(3):418−425.
18. de Vries AL, Doreleijers TA, Steensma TD, Cohen-Kettenis PT. Psychiatric comorbidity in gender dysphoric adolescents. *J Child Psychol Psychiatry.* 2011;52(11):1195−1202.
19. Olson J, Forbes C, Belzer M. Management of the transgender adolescent. *Arch Pediatr Adolesc Med.* 2011;165(2):171−176.
20. Peitzmeier S, Gardner I, Weinand J, Corbet A, Acevedo K. Health impact of chest binding among transgender adults: a community-engaged, cross-sectional study. *Cult Health Sex.* 2017;19(1):64−75.
21. Kosciw J, Greytak E, Giga N, Villenas C, Danischewski D. *The 2015 National School Climate Survey: The Experiences of Lesbian, Gay, Bisexual, Transgender, and Queer Youth in Our Nation's Schools.* New York: NY; 2015.

22. deVries A, Cohen-Kettenis P, Delemarre-Vandewaal H, Holman CW, Goldberg J. *Caring for Transgender Adolescents in BC: Suggested Guidelines*. Vancouver, BC: Trans Care Project; 2006.

23. Safer J, Coleman E, Feldman J, et al. Barriers to health care for transgender individuals. *Curr Opin Endocrinol Diabetes Obes*. 2016;23(2):168–171.

24. Gridley SJ, Crouch JM, Evans Y, et al. Youth and caregiver perspectives on barriers to gender-affirming health care for transgender youth. *J Adolesc Health*. 2016;59(3):254–261.

25. Grant J, Mottet L, Tanis J. *Injustice at Every Turn: A Report of the National Transgender Discrimination Survey*. Washington: DC; 2011.

CHAPTER 3

Puberty

DENNIS M. STYNE, MD

Puberty is not a solitary event but is one stage in the process of development that continues until the end of reproductive life. The hypothalamic–pituitary–gonadal axis is active in the fetus but quiescent during childhood (known as the juvenile pause) until activity increases in the peripubertal period, just before the physical changes of puberty are noted. Increased secretion of pituitary gonadotropins stimulate gonadal sex steroid production which leads to secondary sexual development and the pubertal growth spurt that follows, until ultimately fertility is achieved. The age of menarche has declined over the last 150 years probably due to improvements in socioeconomic conditions, nutrition, and, therefore, the general state of health. However, the age of breast development has decreased to a greater degree than the age of menarche in some substantial studies, and this discrepancy is possibly due to environmental endocrine disruptors since the standard endocrine changes of puberty do not accompany this earlier appearance of breast tissue. These trends toward an earlier onset of thelarche are enhanced due to the effects of the obesity epidemic. Early life adversities have been also associated with earlier menarche. Early menarche (before 11 years) is reported as more common in girl-to-boy sex reassignment applicants than in a control population.

Genetic and exogenous factors can alter age at the onset of puberty. Obesity can decrease the age of onset of puberty in girls, apparently by enhancing breast development due to local aromatase activity in the adipose tissue. Alternatively, a delay in puberty is caused by illness and malnutrition. The age of menarche between mother–daughter pairs reflect the influence of genetic factors. Many genetic loci are identified that are associated with the regulation of menarche and puberty, but no single gene is controlling in normal subjects; some of the associations with pubertal timing are also associated with cancer risk, particularly breast, endometrial, and prostate cancer. In the treatment of transgender youth with gonadotropin-releasing hormone (GnRH) agonist to delay the onset of pubertal development, it is important to consider the familial pattern.

PHYSICAL CHANGES ASSOCIATED WITH PUBERTY

Sexual maturation stages or, as often denoted, "Tanner stages" describe pubertal development in males and females. They allow objective recording of the progression of secondary sexual development. Self-assessment of pubertal development using reference pictures is utilized in clinical or research venues, but this may be less reliable than a physical examination, especially in male puberty assessment or in overweight or obese girls.

Female Changes

Breast development is the first sign of puberty noted by most examiners but an increase in height velocity is closely temporaly associated. Some girls first demonstrate pubic hair appearance before breast development. The first evidence of pubic hair is quite subtle and often requires careful inspection. Breast development (Fig. 3.1A) occurs due to ovarian estrogen secretion, although other hormones are involved. Areolae become more pigmented and erectile, and Montgomery glands at the periphery of the areola appear more prominent as development progresses. Standards are available for the change in areolar (nipple) plateau diameter during puberty but are used more often in research settings than in the clinic. Transient thelarche in which breast development starts earlier than the normal guidelines and then regresses is recognized commonly in some studies; the use of GnRH agonists in early puberty may also lead to regression of breast tissue. Estrogen also causes enlargement of the labia minora and majora, cornification of the vaginal epithelium leading to the dulling of the vaginal mucosa from its prepubertal reddish appearance to pink, and the appearance of a clear or slightly whitish vaginal secretion usually in the months prior to menarche. Pubic hair development

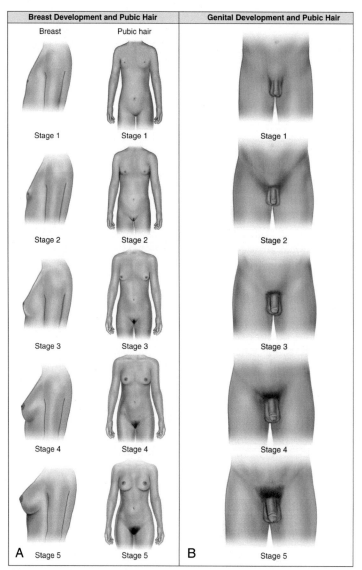

FIG. 3.1 **(A)** Stages of breast development and female pubic hair development, according to Marshall and Tanner. **Stage B1:** Preadolescent; elevation of papilla only. **Stage B2:** Breast bud stage; elevation of breast and papilla as a small mound, and enlargement of areolar diameter. **Stage B3 (not shown):** Further enlargement of breast and areola with no separation of their contours. **Stage B4:** Projection of areola and papilla to form a secondary mound above the level of the breast (not shown). **Stage B5:** Mature stage; projection of papilla only, due to recession of the areola to the general contour of the breast. **Stage P1:** Preadolescent; the vellus over the area is no further developed than that over the anterior abdominal wall (i.e., no pubic hair). **Stage P2:** Sparse growth of long, slightly pigmented, downy hair, straight or only slightly curled, appearing chiefly along the labia. This stage is difficult to see on photographs and is subtle. **Stage P3:** Hair is considerably darker, coarser, and curlier. The hair spreads sparsely over the superior junction of the labia majora. **Stage P4:** Hair is now adult in type, but the area covered by it is still considerably smaller than in most adults. There is no spread to the medial surface of the thighs. **Stage P5:** Hair is adult in quantity and type, distributed as an inverse triangle of the classic feminine pattern. Spread is to the medial surface of the thighs but not up the linea alba or elsewhere above the base of the inverse triangle. **(B)** Stages of male genital development and pubic hair development, according to Marshall and Tanner. Genital: **Stage G1:** Preadolescent. Testes, scrotum, and penis are about the same size and proportion as in early childhood.

(Fig. 3.1B) is caused by adrenal and ovarian androgen secretion. Although usually breast development and growth of pubic hair proceed at similar rates, it is best to stage breast development separately from pubic hair progression since discrepancies occur especially in disease states.

Ultrasonography demonstrates changes in uterine size and shape with pubertal development. The fundus/cervix ratio increases, causing a bulbous appearance to the uterus, and the uterus elongates. An endometrial stripe is an ultrasound feature that appears with the rise in estrogen secretion at the onset of puberty but is not found in premature thelarche. Ovaries also enlarge with pubertal progression. Small cysts are normally present in prepubertal girls and a multicystic appearance develops during puberty, but the pathologic polycystic appearance seen in polycystic ovarian syndrome is not normally present. The developmental stage of the uterus and ovaries is established by comparing these finding with published standards.

Reproductive maturity may occur prior to physical maturity in girls and certainly before psychologic maturity.

Male Changes

An increase in the size of the testes to more than 2.5 cm in the longest diameter, excluding the epididymis, is the first sign of normal puberty in boys: pubertal testes have a volume of 4 mL. This increase in testicular size is mainly due to seminiferous tubular development due to stimulation by follicle-stimulating hormone (FSH), with lesser effect of Leydig cell stimulation by luteinizing hormone (LH). Increased adrenal and testicular androgen secretion cause genital and pubic hair development which should be classified separately in boys as well as girls, as noted in Fig. 3.1. Some suggest ADDING a pubic hair stage 2a (absence of pubic hair

in the presence of a testicular volume of 3 mL or more) to the classic 5 stages of pubertal development as further pubertal development usually soon follows this stage.

As in girls, boys achieve reproductive maturity prior to physical maturity and psychologic maturity.

Age at Onset

The Lawson Wilkins Pediatric Endocrine Society defined the diagnosis of precocious puberty as secondary sexual development starting prior to 6 years in African-American girls and prior to 7 years in Caucasian girls who are otherwise healthy. However, girls with normal body mass index (BMI) values rarely have breast or pubic hair development before 8 years. Since grave diagnoses such as central nervous system (CNS) tumors can cause early puberty, it *is essential to establish that a girl who begins puberty prior to 8 years shows absolutely no signs of neurologic or other conditions that might pathologically advance puberty.*

Boys who are overweight (BMI >85 to <95th percentile for age and gender) tend to have earlier onset of puberty, while obese boys (BMI ≥95th percentile) may start later. However, 9 years is still used as the lower limit of normal pubertal development in males, whereas 14 years is the upper limit of normal development (although 13½ years is used by some SOURCES). Caucasian girls have a mean age of menarche later (12.9 years) than African-American girls (12.3 years).

Delayed onset of pubertal development above the upper age limit of normal may indicate hypothalamic, pituitary, or gonadal failure or, alternatively, normal variation (constitutional delay). The time from the onset of puberty until adult development is complete and is also of importance; significant delays in reaching subsequent stages may indicate any type of hypogonadism.

Stage G2: The scrotum and testes have enlarged, and there is a change in the texture and some reddening of the scrotal skin. There is no enlargement of the penis. **Stage G3:** Growth of the penis has occurred, at first mainly in length but with some increase in breadth; further growth of testes and scrotum. **Stage G4:** Penis further enlarged in length and girth with development of glans. Testes and scrotum further enlarged. The scrotal skin has further darkened. **Stage G5:** Genitalia adult in size and shape. No further enlargement takes place after stage G5 is reached. Pubic hair: **Stage P1:** Preadolescent. The vellus is no further developed than that over the abdominal wall (i.e., no pubic hair). **Stage P2:** Sparse growth of long, slightly pigmented, downy hair, straight or only slightly curled, appearing chiefly at the base of the penis. This is subtle. **Stage P3:** Hair is considerably darker, coarser, and curlier and spreads sparsely. **Stage P4:** Hair is now adult in type, but the area it covers is still considerably smaller than in most adults. There is no spread to the medial surface of the thighs. **Stage P5:** Hair is adult in quantity and type, distributed as an inverse triangle. Spread is to the medial surface of the thighs but not up the linea alba or elsewhere above the base of the inverse triangle. Most men have further spread of pubic hair. (**(A)** and **(B)** Drawings from Styne, *Pediatric Endocrinology: A Clinical Handbook.* Springer International Publishing; 2016, with permission.)

Growth Spurt

The prominent increased growth velocity characteristic of puberty (pubertal growth spurt) is under complex endocrine control. Hypothyroidism decreases or eliminates the pubertal growth spurt. Growth hormone (GH) secretion increases in puberty and causes increased production of insulin-like growth factor. Estrogen, as well as growth hormone, is important in the pubertal growth spurt; when either or both are deficient, the growth spurt is decreased or absent. Estrogen is the most important factor in stimulating maturation of the chondrocytes and osteoblasts, ultimately leading to epiphysial fusion. Estrogen is also of great importance in increasing bone density during puberty.

In girls, the pubertal growth spurt begins in early puberty and is mostly completed by menarche. In boys, the pubertal growth spurt occurs toward the end of puberty, at an average of 2 years later than in girls. A normal boy who is short but appears to have reached only early puberty has a likelihood of significant growth left. The age at onset of the pubertal growth spurt is negatively associated with the BMI in childhood.

Changes in Body Composition

Prepubertal boys and girls start with equal lean body mass, skeletal mass, and body fat, but at maturity, men have approximately 1½ times the lean body mass, skeletal mass, and muscle mass of women, whereas women have twice as much body fat as men. Attainment of peak values of percentage of body fat, lean body mass, and bone mineral density occurs earlier by several years in girls than in boys, as does the earlier peak of height velocity and velocity of weight gain in girls.

Bone accretion mainly occurs during infancy and during puberty. Girls reach peak mineralization between 14 and 16 years of age, whereas boys reach a later peak at 17.5 years; both milestones occur after peak height velocity. Decreased bone mass is found in familial patterns demonstrating the influence of genetic factors. Delayed puberty from any cause including suppression by long-term gonadotropin-releasing hormone agonist therapy for an extended period may cause a significant decrease in bone accretion and a delay in reaching peak bone mineral density. While moderate exercise can increase bone mass, excessive exercise in girls leads to the female athletic triad which is the combination of exercise-induced amenorrhea, premature osteoporosis, and disordered eating/anorexia.

Only a minority of US adolescents receive the recommended daily allowance of calcium (>1000 mg/day depending on age) and vitamin D (400 U), which likely will affect their adult bone health. It is especially important to recommended appropriate calcium and vitamin D intake in teenagers with delayed or absent puberty as well as in patients receiving GnRH agonists.

Other Changes of Puberty

There is extensive change in the anatomy of the brain with pruning of dendritic connections at the beginning of puberty and later increased myelinization of axons. These changes do not cease until at least 25 years of age. The poor judgment and risk-taking behaviors found in early to midpuberty, related to increased dopaminergic activity during this period, contrasts with the maturation of cognitive and executive functions, including judgment, found in later pubertal development, which is related to the later development of the prefrontal cortex. Many significant psychiatric disorders including depression have their onset during puberty. Sleep patterns change during puberty; in the free living state with no light or social cues, adolescents will awaken later (owl-like) than do younger children (lark-like). Then sleep patterns change from "lark-like" to "owl-like" pattern until 19–21 years of age when this change starts to reverse.

PHYSIOLOGY OF PUBERTY

Endocrine Changes From Fetal Life to Puberty

Pituitary gonadotropin secretion is controlled by the hypothalamus, which releases pulses of GnRH into the pituitary-portal system to reach the anterior pituitary gland by 20 weeks of gestation. Control of GnRH secretion is exerted by a *hypothalamic pulse generator* in the arcuate nucleus. It is sensitive to feedback control from sex steroids and inhibin, a gonadal protein product that controls the frequency and amplitude of gonadotropin secretion during development in both sexes and during the progression of menstrual cycle in females.

In males, LH stimulates the Leydig cells to secrete testosterone, and FSH stimulates the Sertoli cells to produce inhibin. Inhibin feeds back on the hypothalamic–pituitary axis to inhibit FSH. In females, FSH stimulates the granulosa cells to produce estrogen and the follicles to secrete inhibin, and LH appears to play a minor role in the endocrine milieu until menarche. With menarche, LH triggers ovulation and later stimulates the theca cells to secrete androgens.

Changes at Birth and the Mini Puberty of INFANCY

At term, serum gonadotropin concentrations are suppressed by maternal estrogen, but with postnatal clearance of high circulating estrogen concentrations, negative inhibition is reduced and postnatal peaks of serum LH and FSH are measurable for several months to up to a few years after birth. While episodic peaks of serum gonadotropins may occur until 2 years of age (mini puberty of infancy), serum gonadotropin concentrations are low during later years in normal childhood. Sex steroids follow this pattern with higher peaks in infancy than childhood.

The Juvenile Pause or the Mid-Childhood Nadir of Gonadotropin Secretion

While serum gonadotropin concentrations are low in mid-childhood, sensitive assays indicate that pulsatile secretion occurs and that the onset of puberty is heralded by an increase in amplitude of secretory events and a change in frequency rather than a de novo appearance of these pulses. Twenty-four-hour mean concentrations of LH, FSH, and testosterone rise measurably within 1 year before the development of physical pubertal changes. Negative feedback inhibition is active during childhood; without sex steroid or inhibin secretion to exert inhibition, serum gonadotropin values are greatly elevated, as might be found in an agonadal individual. During mid-childhood, normal individuals and patients with primary hypogonadism have lower serum gonadotropin levels than they do in the neonatal period, but the range of serum gonadotropin concentrations in primary hypogonadal patients during mid-childhood is still higher than that found in healthy children of the same age. The decrease in serum gonadotropin concentrations in primary agonadal children during mid-childhood has been attributed to an increase in the CNS inhibition of gonadotropin secretion during these years. This inhibition is mediated by γ-aminobutyric acid (GABA) and other inhibitory neuropeptides. The recent discovery of the MRKN3 gene (Makorin Ring Finger Protein 3) which is considered a CNS "brake" on the onset of puberty adds considerably more understanding of the juvenile pause; when this maternally imprinted but paternally expressed gene is silenced, precocious puberty occurs. MRNK3 mutations occur in 46% of familial precocious puberty cases to date. More recently, inactivating mutations of the Delta-like 1 homolog (DLK1) gene which is also expressed only in the father were found in girls with precocious

puberty. Thus, the juvenile pause in normal children and those with primary gonadal failure appears to be due to CNS restraint of GnRH secretion.

Peripubertal Gonadotropin Increase

Before the onset of puberty there is a circadian rhythm of low amplitude secretion of LH and FSH. Thus the endocrine changes of puberty build on preexisting patterns of hypothalamic pituitary hormone secretion. As puberty begins, the secretion of GnRH increases both in amplitude and frequency first in the early hours of sleep. LH and FSH values rise in response. A few hours after the gonadotropin peaks serum testosterone and estrogen concentrations rise demonstrating the biosynthesis of sex steroids and aromatization of testosterone to estrogen. Thus puberty is characterized by increased amplitude of peaks of gonadotropins compared to the prepubertal period. The peaks of serum LH and FSH occur more often during waking hours with the progression of puberty. As reproductive maturation is achieved in late puberty gonadotropin and sex steroid peaks occur throughout the day, and there is no longer a circadian rhythm.

During the peripubertal period of endocrine changes prior to secondary sexual development, gonadotropin secretion becomes less sensitive to negative feedback inhibition. An equilibrium-balancing pubertal concentration of gonadotropins and sex steroids is reached, but at the onset of puberty, both gonadotropins and sex steroid concentrations remain at low levels which require sensitive assays to detect.

Several neurotransmitters are invoked in bringing about the onset of puberty, including GABA and N-methyl-D-aspartate. KISS1, a human metastasis suppressor gene at locus 19p13.3, codes for kisspeptin, an important agent in the process. Kisspeptin is the agonist for GPR54 (previously called kisspeptin receptor), a Gq/11-coupled receptor of the rhodopsin family (metastin receptor), found in the brain, mainly in the hypothalamus and basal ganglia and the placenta. KISS1 mRNA levels rise with the onset of puberty in male and female monkeys as they develop from the juvenile to the midpubertal stage. When kisspeptin is infused into the brain GnRH-primed juvenile female rhesus monkeys, GnRH is secreted, while if GnRH antagonists are also infused, no GnRH is secreted. Thus it appears that KISS1 exerts its effects through the GPR54 receptor of the primate hypothalamus and that at the end of the juvenile pause, this signaling contributes to the pubertal increase in pulsatile GnRH secretion. A decrease in expression of MKRN3, considered to act as a CNS brake on pubertal development, occurs at the time of puberty. Familial precocious puberty, passed down through the father occurs with a decreased expression of this imprinted gene.

Highly sensitive immunoradiometric and immuno-chemiluminometric assays "third-generation assays" and now high-performance liquid chromatography (HPLC)—tandem mass spectroscopy for gonadotropin determination are sensitive enough to indicate the onset of pubertal development with single basal samples usually eliminating the need to perform GnRH or GnRH agonist testing. Basal LH values in the pubertal range according to the laboratory reference ranges for the laboratory being utilized in a child with early sexual development indicate the onset of central precocious puberty or in an older child of normal puberty as they are highly predictive of elevated peak GnRH-stimulated LH. Values are laboratory specific, but LH results over 0.3 mIU/mL are considered indicative of pubertal development. Once the LH secretion increases at the onset of puberty in boys, there is a significant rise in testosterone secretion as the testicular volume increases from a prepubertal volume of 1−2 mL to pubertal volumes equal to or exceeding 4 mL and extending up to 25 mL. As with LH and FSH determinations, testosterone must be measured by a laboratory that performs highly sensitive and specific assays, usually by HPLC followed by tandem mass spectroscopy, with the results compared to age- and pubertal-stage-appropriate standards. To repeat, standard LH, FSH, and testosterone assays are not sensitive enough to detect the changes seen in early pubertal development. Just requesting LH, FSH, or testosterone determinations frequently leads to the performance of less-sensitive assays used in adults. Pediatric assays are usually indicated on order menus as such.

Sex Steroid Secretion

Sex steroid secretion is temporally associated with the development of gonadotropin secretion. During the postnatal period of increased episodic gonadotropin secretion, plasma concentrations of gonadal steroids also rise indicating the functional stimulatory ability of the newborn gonad. During the middle childhood period of relatively suppressed gonadotropin secretion (the juvenile pause), gonadal stimulatory activity decreases as well. However, repeated administration of human chorionic gonadotrophin can stimulate the testes to secrete testosterone. There is a low level of

ovarian secretory activity in girls demonstrated by measurable estradiol levels in sensitive assays. Serum gonadal steroid concentrations progressively increase with the onset of puberty along with increasing gonadotropin concentrations. Although values vary by laboratory, a prepubertal value of estradiol less than 16 pg/mL (58.7 pmol/L) or a testosterone value of less than 8 ng/dL (0.3 nmol/L) are general guidelines for prepubertal values. Although gonadal sex steroids are secreted in a diurnal rhythm in early puberty, sex steroids are bound to sex hormone—binding globulin (SHBG or TeBG), leading to a longer half-life of sex steroids compared to gonadotropins. Because of this, random measurement of gonadal sex steroids can be used to determine pubertal staging more than random measurements of serum gonadotropins. In spite of that, there is a considerable variation in estradiol secretion so that early pubertal girls may or may not have pubertal values of estradiol on any given sample.

Most (97%−99%) of the circulating estradiol and testosterone is associated with SHBG. Prepubertal boys and girls have equal concentrations of SHBG, but adult males have only half the concentration of SHBG compared with adult females since testosterone decreases SHBG and estrogen increases SHBG. Lower SHBG levels in males amplify the effect of androgens in men. Adult men have 20 times the amount of plasma testosterone compared to adult women; however, adult men have 40 times the amount of free testosterone than adult women.

Sex steroid treatment may be started in the course of treatment of appropriate patients after pubertal suppression in the treatment of gender dysphoria.

Gonadotropin-Releasing Hormone Stimulation

GnRH has been used as a test of pubertal development. Response, primarily in LH, to exogenous GnRH changes with age. Native GnRH is not available clinically, so the use of GnRH agonists has been used for such testing as well as for treatment in pubertal suppression. If GnRH agonist is administered to children younger than 2 years of age, pituitary secretion of LH and FSH increases in a manner similar to pubertal children due to the mini puberty of infancy. Later during the juvenile pause, when endogenous GnRH secretion has decreased, GnRH agonist exerts less effect on LH release. When puberty begins, administration of the GnRH agonist again brings about a higher peak of LH concentration in boys and girls, and this response continues until adulthood. While there is no change in peak FSH secretion after GnRH agonist with the onset of puberty, there is a greater release of FSH in females compared to males at all stages.

Reference ranges of the LH concentration at different stages of puberty vary between laboratories, but, in general, if the basal concentration of plasma LH rises above 0.3 or the plasma concentration of peak LH is over 5.5 U/L, 1 hour after 10 μg/kg of subcutaneous GnRH or GnRH agonist administration, the endocrine changes of puberty had begun. More specifically, it is reported that when boys have, after 10 μg/kg of leuprolide acetate, a 4-h LH value over 14.8−15 units per liter, puberty has begun.

Endogenous GnRH is secreted episodically about every 90−120 min in response to the CNS *pulse generator, and gonadotropin secretion follows in a pulsatile fashion.* Exogenous GnRH can be used to stimulate pubertal gonadotropin secretion when it is administered to patients in episodic boluses by a programmable pump program to reflect the natural secretory episodes of GnRH. After only a few days of exogenously administered GnRH boluses, a prepubertal subject without initial significant gonadotropin peaks will have reached a normal pubertal pattern of episodic secretion of gonadotropins. Patients who have no or inadequate gonadotropin secretion to progress through reproductive development may reach a pattern of normal adult episodic gonadotropin secretion by this method of administration of pulsatile GnRH administration. This phenomenon is used in clinical practice to bring about ovulation or spermatogenesis to foster fertility.

Alternatively, if GnRH is administered continuously rather than in pulses, a brief period of increased gonadotropin secretion is followed by LH and FSH suppression. This phenomenon in which continuous GnRH secretion ultimately decreases the number and activity of the GnRH receptors was utilized in the development of GnRH agonists. These agonists act as a long-term continuous infusion of GnRH which suppresses gonadotropin secretion and thereby suppresses gonadal steroid secretion. It is this phenomenon that is utilized in treatment with GnRH analogs for therapeutic effect in conditions such as central precocious puberty and endometriosis, and can bring about a chemical test castration in men with prostatic carcinoma. It is the suppressive action of GnRH agonist on pubertal progression that is utilized in the delaying of pubertal development in gender dysphoria as discussed elsewhere in this volume.

Leptin and Puberty

Leptin, produced in adipose cells, can suppress appetite when it interacts with its receptor in the hypothalamus. Leptin plays a major role in pubertal development in mice and rats but has a modified role in human puberty. An extremely obese leptin-deficient girl aged 9 years had a bone age of 13 years which is compatible with the onset of normal puberty. She had no significant gonadotropin pulsatility and no secondary sexual development of puberty. After recombinant DNA-derived leptin was administrated to her, she began to demonstrate gonadotropin peaks, estrogen secretion increased, and secondary sexual development occurred. Individuals who are leptin resistant due to leptin receptor deficiency or abnormality will also have disorders of puberty. Leptin does not appear to trigger the onset of puberty in normal adolescents as changes in plasma leptin concentrations accompany pubertal changes rather than precede them. Leptin is necessary but not sufficient for pubertal development.

Ovulation and Menarche

Positive feedback of estrogen on the hypothalamic−pituitary axis is a late development during puberty and is the phenomenon that allows ovulation and menarche. Menarche usually follows thelarche by 2.5−3 years. After midpuberty, estrogen in the appropriate amount at the appropriate time can stimulate gonadotropin release, whereas higher doses of estrogen will still suppress gonadotropin secretion. The ratio of LH to FSH secretion rises as the frequency of pulsatile GnRH release increases during the late follicular phase of the normal menstrual cycle. Increased LH secretion stimulates estrogen production from the ovary which through positive feedback leads to the midcycle LH surge that causes ovulation. As discussed above, administration of GnRH in pulsatile fashion by a programmable pump is utilized to allow fertility in patients with hypogonadotropic hypogonadism or hypothalamic GnRH deficiency as this pump can mimic the natural pattern of gonadotropin secretion and trigger ovulation.

However, even if the midcycle surge of gonadotropins is present, ovulation may not occur during the first menstrual cycles after menarche as 90% of menstrual cycles are anovulatory in the first year after menarche. By 5 years after menarche, about 80% of periods are ovulatory. The high prevalence of anovulatory periods during this period, however, may be less due to development than unrecognized polycystic ovary syndrome. However, it is always important to realize that some of the first cycles after menarche may be ovulatory, and fertility is possible in the first cycle.

Adrenarche

Understanding of the control of adrenal androgen secretion is incomplete. The adrenal cortex normally secretes the weak androgens dehydroepiandrosterone (DHEA), its sulfate—dehydroepiandrosterone sulfate (DHEAS), and androstenedione in increasing amounts beginning at about 6–7 years of age in girls and 7–8 years of age in boys. This is several years before the appearance of pubic hair or acne. A continued rise in adrenal androgen secretion persists until late puberty in normal individuals. Adrenarche is the onset of the secretion of adrenal androgens, pubarche is the appearance of pubic hair or acne or comedones, while gonadarche is the secretion of gonadal sex steroids. Adrenarche precedes gonadarche by several years in a normal individual. The age at adrenarche does not usually influence age at gonadarche. Furthermore, since GnRH agonist can only inhibit gonadotropin secretion, patients treated with a GnRH agonist progress through adrenarche despite their suppressed gonadarche.

DELAYED PUBERTY OR ABSENT PUBERTY (SEXUAL INFANTILISM)

Any girl of 13 years or boy of 14 years (13.5 years in some sources) of age without signs of pubertal development falls more than 2.5 standard deviations (SDs) above the mean and is considered to have delayed puberty. It is important to determine which of these patients older than these guidelines have constitutionally delayed puberty and which have organic disease. A patient wishing gender reassignment who has either of these diagnoses will not need GnRH agonist therapy at the average age of puberty.

Constitutional Delay in Growth and Adolescence

Constitutional delay in puberty should be considered the diagnosis in a patient with delayed onset of secondary sexual development, whose stature is shorter than that of age-matched peers but who consistently maintains a normal growth velocity for bone age and whose skeletal development is delayed more than 2 SDs from the mean, especially if there is a family history of a similar pattern of development in a parent or sibling. These patients are at the older end of the normal distribution curve describing the age at onset of puberty. At the time of examination, the initial elevation of gonadal sex steroids may have already begun, even if the patient shows no physical signs of puberty and their basal LH concentrations measured by ultrasensitive third-generation assays or their plasma LH response to intravenous GnRH or GnRH agonist is pubertal. Boys who have an 8-a.m serum testosterone value above 20 ng/dL (0.7 mmol/L) are likely to begin secondary sexual development within a period of 15 months.

In some cases, observation for endocrine or physical signs of puberty must continue for a period of months or years before the diagnosis is made. While signs of puberty appear after the patient reaches a skeletal age of 11 years (girls) or 12 years (boys), in general, there is great variation. By 18 years of chronologic age, most patients with constitutional delay in adolescence will have secondary sexual development. Adrenarche is reported to be delayed—along with gonadarche—in constitutional delay in puberty. Constitutional delay is a diagnosis of exclusion and pathologic etiologies of delayed puberty must be considered before this diagnosis is made.

Hypogonadotropic Hypogonadism

The absent or decreased ability of the hypothalamus to secrete GnRH or of the pituitary gland to secrete LH and FSH characterizes hypogonadotropic hypogonadism. If the pituitary deficiency is limited to gonadotropins, a patient's stature is usually close to average height for age until the usual age of the pubertal growth spurt, in contrast to shorter patients with constitutional delay. However, if GH deficiency accompanies gonadotropin deficiency, severe short stature will result.

Central nervous system disorders

Tumors. A CNS tumor involving the hypothalamus or pituitary gland can interfere with hypothalamic–pituitary–gonadal function as well as control of GH, adrenocorticotropic hormone, thyrotropin, prolactin, and vasopressin secretion; the patient with acquired anterior and posterior pituitary deficiencies is likely to have a serious problem such as a CNS tumor. It is imperative that a hypothalamic–pituitary tumor be eliminated as the cause of delayed puberty before assigning another diagnosis such as constitutional delay.

Other acquired central nervous system disorders.

Infiltrative lesions, tuberculous or sarcoid granulomas, other postinfectious inflammatory lesions, vascular lesions, and trauma may cause hypogonadotropic hypogonadism.

Developmental defects. Developmental defects of the CNS may cause hypogonadotropic hypogonadism or other types of hypothalamic dysfunction. Cleft palate or other midline anomalies may also be associated with hypothalamic dysfunction.

Radiation therapy. CNS radiation therapy involving the hypothalamic—pituitary area can lead to hypogonadotropic hypogonadism. However, GH is more frequently affected than gonadotropin secretion. Other hypothalamic deficiencies such as gonadotropin deficiency, hypothyroidism, and hyperprolactinemia occur more often with higher doses of radiation.

Isolated gonadotropin deficiency

Kallmann syndrome is the most common genetic form of isolated gonadotropin deficiency. Gonadotropin deficiency in these patients is associated with hypoplasia or aplasia of the olfactory lobes and olfactory bulb causing hyposmia or anosmia. This is a familial syndrome of variable manifestations in which anosmia may occur with or without hypogonadism in a given member of a kindred. *X-linked Kallmann syndrome* is due to gene deletions in the region of Xp22.3, causing the absence of the *KAL1* gene which codes for anosmin, an adhesion molecule that plays a key role in the migration of GnRH neurons and olfactory nerves to the hypothalamus. Adult height is normal, although patients experience delays reaching adult height. *Kallmann syndrome 2* is inherited in an autosomal dominant pattern and is due to a mutation in the *FGFR1* (*fibroblast growth factor receptor 1*) gene. *Kallmann syndrome 3* exhibits an autosomal recessive pattern and appears to be related to mutations in *PROKR2* and *PROK2*, encoding prokineticin receptor-2 and prokineticin-2, respectively. FGF8 may also be involved.

While kisspeptin and G protein—coupled receptor 54 (GRP54) play important roles at the onset of puberty, only rare patients have been reported with defects in the kisspeptin—GPR54 axis due to a loss of functional mutation in the gene for the GRP54 receptor. Mutations of the *GnRH receptor* gene, *GnRHR*, were noted many years ago, and more recently, mutations in the *GnRH1* gene has been demonstrated. Other mutations causing hypogonadotropic hypogonadism without anosmia include the *GPR54*, *SF-1* (*steroidogenic factor 1*), *HESX-1* (*Hesx-1 homeodomain*), *LHX3* (*LIM homeobox gene 3*), and *PROP-1* (*prophet of PIT1*) genes. X-linked congenital adrenal hypoplasia

is associated with hypogonadotropic hypogonadism. Adrenal hypoplasia congenital (AHC), glycerol kinase deficiency, and muscular dystrophy have also been linked to this syndrome. The gene locus is at Xp21.3-p21.2 and involves a mutation in the *DAX1* gene in many but not all patients.

Idiopathic hypopituitary dwarfism (growth hormone deficiency in the absence of defined anatomic or organic defects)

Patients with congenital GH deficiency have early onset of growth failure; this feature distinguishes them from patients with GH deficiency due to hypothalamic tumors, who usually have late onset of growth failure. Even without associated gonadotropin deficiency, untreated GH-deficient patients often have delayed onset of puberty associated with their delayed bone ages. Idiopathic hypopituitarism is usually sporadic but may follow an autosomal recessive or X-linked inheritance pattern due to one of the gene defects listed earlier.

Miscellaneous disorders

Several genetic conditions including Prader—Willi syndrome and *Bardet—Biedl syndrome combine syndromic physical findings with delayed/absent pubertal development.*

Chronic disease and malnutrition. A delay in sexual maturation may be due to chronic disease or malnutrition. Weight loss to less than 80% of ideal body weight, caused by disease or voluntary dieting, may result in gonadotropin deficiency; weight gain toward the ideal usually restores gonadotropin function, but there is often a delay after the weight gain.

Celiac disease can be found in approximately 1% of the general population but in about 10% of type I diabetes patients. This immunological disorder of gluten intolerance produces numerous clinical sequelae, including late puberty, poor growth, delayed menarche, and osteopenia.

Anorexia nervosa. Anorexia nervosa involves weight loss associated with a psychologic disorder and carries a significant risk of mortality. This condition usually affects girls who develop a disturbed body image and exhibit typical behavior such as avoidance of food and induction of regurgitation after ingestion; boys may be affected as well. Weight loss may be so severe as to cause fatal complications such as immune dysfunction, fluid and electrolyte imbalance, or circulatory collapse. Primary or secondary amenorrhea is a classic finding in affected girls and has been correlated with the degree of weight loss, although there is evidence that patients with anorexia nervosa may cease to menstruate before their substantial weight loss is exhibited. Prepubertal gonadotropin values, impaired monthly cycles of gonadotropin secretion, and retention of a prepubertal diurnal rhythm of gonadotropin secretion are found in anorexia nervosa patients, patterns that indicate a reversion to an earlier stage of the endocrine changes of puberty.

Increased physical activity. Strenuous athletics and ballet dancing taken to the extreme may lead to the female athletic triad of delayed menarche, irregular or absent menstrual periods and decreased bone density. The amenorrhea may be caused by the increased physical activity rather than decreased weight, as some amenorrheic girls may resume menses while temporarily bedridden even though their weight does not yet change.

Hypothyroidism. Hypothyroidism can delay all aspects of growth and maturation, including puberty and menarche. With thyroxine therapy, catch-up growth and resumed pubertal development and menses occur.

Hypergonadotropic Hypogonadism

Primary gonadal failure characterized by elevated gonadotropin concentrations due to the absence of negative feedback effects of gonadal sex steroids and inhibin is called hypergonadotropic hypogonadism. The most common causes are chromosomal abnormalities which are usually associated with somatic abnormalities as in the syndrome of seminiferous tubule dysgenesis (Klinefelter syndrome classically 47XXY) and the syndrome of gonadal dysgenesis (Turner syndrome classically 46X), although isolated gonadal failure can also present with delayed puberty without other physical findings.

PRECOCIOUS PUBERTY (SEXUAL PRECOCITY)

All sources agree that the appearance of secondary sexual development before the age of 9 years in boys is precocious puberty. However, there remains controversy over the lower limits of normal in girls. The Pediatric Endocrine Society accepted that the appearance of secondary sexual development before the age of 7 years in Caucasian girls and 6 years in African-American girls constitutes precocious sexual development, but others remain concerned that pubertal development between 7 and 8 years for Caucasian and 6 and 8 years for African-American girls indicates a pathological state.

Thus, if a girl has the onset of puberty before 8 years, especially when there is no overweight or obesity, one must have a high index of suspicion for pathology. The child must have absolutely no sign of CNS disorder or other possible cause that might trigger pathologic precocious puberty. A careful search for historical or physical features of organic disease must occur before a girl with precocious puberty between 6 and 8 years is considered normal. When the cause of precocious puberty is premature activation of the hypothalamic–pituitary axis, and the condition is gonadotropin dependent, the diagnosis is *central (complete or true) precocious puberty*; if ectopic gonadotropin secretion occurs in boys or autonomous sex steroid secretion occurs in either sex, the condition is not gonadotropin dependent, and the diagnosis is peripheral or *incomplete precocious puberty*. In all forms of sexual precocity, there is an increase in growth velocity, somatic development, and skeletal maturation. This rapid skeletal development leads to tall stature during childhood and the paradox of the tall child growing up to become a short adult because of early epiphysial fusion.

Central (Complete or True) Precocious Puberty

Idiopathic central (complete or true) isosexual precociious puberty. Affected children, with no familial tendency toward early development and no organic disease, may be considered to have idiopathic central isosexual precocious puberty. Pubertal development may follow the normal course or may wax and wane. Serum gonadotropin and sex steroid concentrations and response to GnRH or GnRH agonists are similar to those found in normal pubertal subjects. Girls present with idiopathic central precocious puberty more commonly than boys.

Genetic causes of central precocious puberty. The *MRKN3* gene is maternally imprinted, leading to silencing of the maternal allele, but the paternal allele is active. This gene is considered to exert a braking effect on pubertal development, and thus, when a paternal inactivating mutation occurs, since the maternal allele is already silenced, the child experiences precocious puberty. Defects in the DLK1 gene which is also paternally inherited can also lead to precocious puberty.

1. *CNS disorders.* CNS tumors are more common causes of central precocious puberty in boys than in girls, so a high index of suspicion is essential. Optic gliomas or hypothalamic gliomas, astrocytomas, ependymomas, germinomas, and other CNS tumors may cause precocious puberty by interfering with the

neural pathways that inhibit GnRH secretion, thus releasing the CNS restraint of gonadotropin secretion. Central precocious puberty is usually amenable to treatment with GnRH agonists once the underlying CNS condition is resolved.

Peripheral or Incomplete Isosexual Precocious Puberty

If puberty does not emanate from pulsatile secretion of GnRH from the CNS, the child has peripheral or incomplete precocious puberty. In all cases, sex steroids are elevated and gonadotropins are suppressed by the sex steroids.

1. *Peripheral or incomplete isosexual precocious puberty in genotypic males.* Premature sexual development in the absence of hypothalamic–pituitary maturation may occur in males from either: (1) ectopic or autonomous endogenous secretion of hCG or LH or iatrogenic administration of human chorionic gonatotropin (hCG), which can stimulate Leydig cell production of testosterone or (2) autonomous endogenous secretion of androgens from the testes or adrenal glands or from iatrogenic exogenous administration of androgens. (In females, secretion of hCG does not by itself cause secondary sexual development.)

Peripheral or incomplete isosexual precocious puberty in genotypic females. Females with peripheral isosexual precocity have a source of excessive estrogens which may occur due to autonomous estrogen secretion from the ovary or more rarely the adrenal gland or from exogenous estrogen administration.

Variations of Puberty

Premature thelarche. The term *premature thelarche* denotes unilateral or bilateral breast enlargement without other signs of androgen or estrogen secretion. Patients are usually younger than 3 years; the breast enlargement may regress within months or remain until actual pubertal development occurs at a normal age. Areolar development and vaginal mucosal signs of estrogen effect are usually absent or minimal. Premature thelarche may be caused by brief episodes of estrogen secretion from ovarian cysts. Plasma estrogen levels are usually low in this disorder, perhaps because blood samples are characteristically drawn after the initiating secretory event.

Premature adrenarche. Premature adrenarche is the early onset of adrenal androgen production which leads to premature pubarche which is the early appearance of pubic or axillary hair without other significant signs of virilization or puberty. This condition allows the secondary sexual development of puberty to occur at the normal age for puberty. It is not progressive. Premature adrenarche is usually found in children older than 6 years and is more common in girls than in boys. Plasma DHEAS levels are generally elevated to stage 2 pubertal levels, higher than normally found in this age group but well below those seen with adrenal tumors.

1. *Adolescent gynecomastia.* Transient unilateral or bilateral gynecomastia occurs in up to 75% of boys, usually beginning in stage 2 or 3 of puberty and regressing about 2 years later. Serum estrogen and testosterone concentrations are normal. Some severely affected patients with extremely prominent breast development may require reduction mammoplasty if psychologic distress is extreme, but reassurance is usually all that is required.

Klinefelter syndrome and the syndromes of incomplete androgen resistance are also associated with gynecomastia and must be differentiated from the gynecomastia of normal pubertal development in males. Certain medications list gynecomastia as a side effect. Marijuana use can also elevate the risk for the gynecomastia.

FURTHER READING

1. Abreu AP, Dauber A, Macedo DB, et al. Central precocious puberty caused by mutations in the imprinted gene MKRN3. *N Engl J Med.* 2013;368(26):2467–2475. https://doi.org/10.1056/NEJMoa1302160.
2. Albrecht L, Styne D. Laboratory testing of gonadal steroids in children. *Pediatr Endocrinol Rev.* 2007;5(suppl 1): 599–607.
3. Bayley N, Pinneau SR. Tables for predicting adult height from skeletal age: revised for use with the Greulich-Pyle hand standards. *J Pediatr.* 1952;40(4):423–441.
4. Busch AS, Hagen CP, Almstrup K, Juul A. Circulating MKRN3 levels decline during puberty in healthy boys. *J Clin Endocrinol Metab.* 2016;101(6):2588–2593. https://doi.org/10.1210/jc.2016-1488.
5. Carel JC, Eugster EA, Rogol A, et al. Consensus statement on the use of gonadotropin-releasing hormone analogs in children. *Pediatrics.* 2009;123(4):e752–e762. https://doi.org/10.1542/peds.2008-1783.
6. Davenport ML. Approach to the patient with Turner syndrome. *J Clin Endocrinol Metab.* 2010;95(4): 1487–1495. https://doi.org/10.1210/jc.2009-0926.
7. de Vries AL, Klink D, Cohen-Kettenis PT. What the primary care pediatrician needs to know about gender incongruence and gender dysphoria in children and adolescents. *Pediatr Clin North Am.* 2016;63(6):1121–1135. https://doi.org/10.1016/j.pcl.2016.07.011.

8. Finlayson CA, Styne DM, Jameson JL, De Groot LJ, eds. *Endocrinology: Adult and Pediatric.* 7th ed. Philadelphia, PA: Elsevier; 2015.

9. Greulich WW, Pyle SI. *Radiographic Atlas of Skeletal Development of the Hand and Wrist.* 2nd ed. Stanford. CA: Stanford University Press; 1959.

10. Harrington J, Palmert MR. Clinical review: distinguishing constitutional delay of growth and puberty from isolated hypogonadotropic hypogonadism: critical appraisal of available diagnostic tests. *J Clin Endocrinol Metab.* 2012; 97(9):3056–3067. https://doi.org/10.1210/jc.2012-1598.

11. Hembree WC, Cohen-Kettenis PT, Gooren L, et al. Endocrine treatment of gender-dysphoric/gender-incongruent persons: an endocrine society clinical practice guideline. *J Clin Endocrinol Metab.* 2017;102(11):3869–3903. https://doi.org/10.1210/jc.2017-01658.

12. Herman-Giddens ME, Slora EJ, Wasserman RC, et al. Secondary sexual characteristics and menses in young girls seen in office practice: a study from the pediatric research in office settings network. *Pediatrics.* 1997;99(4): 505–512.

13. Herman-Giddens ME, Steffes J, Harris D, et al. Secondary sexual characteristics in boys: data from the pediatric research in office settings network. *Pediatrics.* 2012;130(5): e1058–e1068. https://doi.org/10.1542/peds.2011-3291.

14. Himes JH, Park K, Styne D. Menarche and assessment of body mass index in adolescent girls. *J Pediatr.* 2009;155(3): 393–397. https://doi.org/10.1016/j.jpeds.2009.03.036.

15. Hughes IA. Releasing the brake on puberty. *N Engl J Med.* 2013;368(26):2513–2515. https://doi.org/10.1056/NEJMe 1306743.

16. Kaplowitz PB, Oberfield SE. Reexamination of the age limit for defining when puberty is precocious in girls in the United States: implications for evaluation and treatment. Drug and Therapeutics and Executive Committees of the Lawson Wilkins Pediatric Endocrine Society. *Pediatrics.* 1999;104(4 Pt 1):936–941.

17. Kuohung W, Kaiser UB. GPR54 and KiSS-1: role in the regulation of puberty and reproduction. *Rev Endocr Metab Disord.* 2006;7(4):257–263. https://doi.org/10.1007/ s11154-006-9020-2.

18. Latronico AC, Brito VN, Carel JC. Causes, diagnosis, and treatment of central precocious puberty. *Lancet Diabetes Endocrinol.* 2016;4(3):265–274. https://doi.org/10.1016/ s2213-8587(15)00380-0.

19. Lee JM, Wasserman R, Kaciroti N, et al. Timing of puberty in overweight versus obese boys. *Pediatrics.* 2016;137(2): e20150164. https://doi.org/10.1542/peds.2015-0164.

20. Lee Y, Styne D. Influences on the onset and tempo of puberty in human beings and implications for adolescent psychological development. *Horm Behav.* 2013;64(2): 250–261. https://doi.org/10.1016/j.yhbeh.2013.03.014.

21. Livadas S, Chrousos GP. Control of the onset of puberty. *Curr Opin Pediatr.* 2016;28(4):551–558. https://doi.org/ 10.1097/.

22. Loomba-Albrecht LA, Styne DM. Effect of puberty on body composition. *Curr Opin Endocrinol Diabetes Obes.* 2009; 16(1):10–15.

23. Marshall WA, Tanner JM. Variations in pattern of pubertal changes in girls. *Arch Dis Child.* 1969;44(235):291–303.

24. Marshall WA, Tanner JM. Variations in the pattern of pubertal changes in boys. *Arch Dis Child.* 1970;45(239): 13–23.

25. Palmert MR, Dunkel L. Clinical practice. Delayed puberty. *N Engl J Med.* 2012;366(5):443–453. https://doi.org/ 10.1056/NEJMcp1109290.

26. Rosenfield RL, Cooke DW, Radovick S. Puberty and its disorders in the female. In: Sperling MA, ed. *Pediatric Endocrinology.* 4th ed. Philadelphia, PA: Elsevier; 2014: 569–663.

27. Rosenfield RL, Lipton RB, Drum ML. Thelarche, pubarche, and menarche attainment in children with normal and elevated body mass index. *Pediatrics.* 2009;123(1): 84–88. https://doi.org/10.1542/peds.2008-0146.

28. Tanaka T, Niimi H, Matsuo N, et al. Results of long-term follow-up after treatment of central precocious puberty with leuprorelin acetate: evaluation of effectiveness of treatment and recovery of gonadal function. The TAP-144-SR Japanese Study Group on Central Precocious Puberty. *J Clin Endocrinol Metab.* 2005;90(3):1371–1376. https://doi.org/10.1210/jc.2004-1863.

29. Styne DM. *Puberty in Pediatric Endocrinology: A Clinical Handbook.* Switzerland: Springer International Publishing; 2016:189–233.

30. Styne DM, Grumbach MM. Puberty: ontogeny, neuroendocrinology, physiology, and disorders. In: Melmed S, Polonsky KS, Larsen PR, Kronenberg HM, eds. *Williams Textbook of Endocrinology.* 12th ed. Philadelphia, PA: Saunders, Elsevier; 2015.

31. Voutilainen R, Jaaskelainen J. Premature adrenarche: etiology, clinical findings, and consequences. *J Steroid Biochem Mol Biol.* 2015;145:226–236. https://doi.org/10.1016/ j.jsbmb.2014.06.004.

32. Wolf RM, Long D. Pubertal development. *Pediatr Rev.* 2016;37(7):292–300. https://doi.org/10.1542/pir.2015-0065.

CHAPTER 4

GnRH Analogs (Mechanism, Past Studies, Drug Options, Use in Precocious Puberty, Use in Gender-Nonconforming Youth)

ANISHA GOHIL, DO • ERICA A. EUGSTER, MD

HISTORICAL PERSPECTIVE

The history that led to the discovery and development of gonadotropin-releasing hormone analogs (GnRHas) is a fascinating one. Gregor Popa and Una Fielding discovered the hypophyseal portal system in 1930, originally describing this network of blood vessels in the rat.[1,2] In 1937, Geoffrey Harris demonstrated that the anterior pituitary was controlled by the central nervous system, and his later research in the 1940s and 1950s showed specifically that this control came from the hypothalamus via the hypophyseal portal system.[1–3] In 1971, Schally et al. discovered that one polypeptide, gonadotropin-releasing hormone (GnRH), when isolated from porcine hypothalami stimulated the release of follicle-stimulating hormone (FSH) and luteinizing hormone (LH) from the pituitary gland across species. They not only identified the structure of this polypeptide but also created a synthetic form of it that exhibited the same downstream effects.[4] Roger Guilleman worked independently in a competitive race with Andrew Schally in the discovery of hypothalamic regulatory hormones.[1,5] In 1977, both were awarded the Nobel Prize in Physiology or Medicine for their scientific discoveries.[6] A more refined physiological understanding of GnRH was attained in 1978 when Belchetz discovered that the pattern of GnRH delivery affected gonadotropin secretion. Intermittent administration stimulated gonadotropin secretion while constant administration resulted in a paradoxical downregulation of the hypothalamic–pituitary–gonadal (HPG) axis.[7] It was this seminal discovery that paved the way for the development of the GnRHas and their subsequent utilization in the clinical arena.

In the following years, potential applications of GnRHas were investigated in numerous clinical settings, including central precocious puberty (CPP), female and male contraception, endometriosis, uterine fibroids, polycystic ovarian disease, hirsutism, menstrual cycle disorders, prostate cancer, and assisted fertilization.[6,8] GnRHas transformed the treatment of CPP since their first reported use in 1981 and quickly became the standard of care for this condition. By 1993, three different GnRHas—leuprolide, nafarelin, and histrelin—had each received the Food and Drug Administration's (FDA) approval for the treatment of CPP. The initial routes of administration were restricted to intranasal and subcutaneous, both of which required daily dosing.[9] Subsequently, a depot form of leuprolide was developed that allowed for monthly intramuscular administration, and additional extended-release formulations of GnRHas continue to emerge.[9–11] Currently, 3-monthly intramuscular injections, 6-monthly intramuscular injections, and yearly subcutaneous implants are also available.[12,13] Intramuscular preparations have also been administered subcutaneously with good success by some providers (personal communication).

The use of GnRHas to block puberty and suppress the HPG axis in patients with gender dysphoria is associated with improved physical and psychological outcomes.[14] Following the first published case of the successful use of the GnRHa, triptorelin, in a female-to-male (FTM) individual in 1998, this class of medications became established as the treatment of choice for pubertal suppression in the gender dysphoric patient.[14–16] Fig. 4.1 illustrates a historical timeline of the discovery of

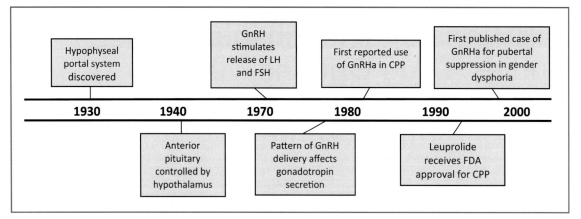

FIG. 4.1 Timeline of significant landmarks in the history of gonadotropin-releasing hormone (*GnRH*) analogs (*GnRHas*). *CPP*, central precocious puberty; *FDA*, Food and Drug Administration; *FSH*, follicle-stimulating hormone; *LH*, luteinizing hormone.

GnRH and the clinical use of GnRHas in pediatric patients throughout the past century.

PHYSIOLOGY AND MECHANISM OF ACTION

GnRH is synthesized in the hypothalamus and secreted into the hypophyseal portal system where it travels to the anterior pituitary. Here it acts at the GnRH receptor to stimulate the release of LH and FSH from the gonadotrope cells. The gonadotropins act on the ovary and testis to stimulate production of sex steroids, which in turn leads to the development of secondary sexual characteristics. Sex steroids exert regulatory positive and negative feedback at the level of the hypothalamus and pituitary.[8,17,18]

Pulsatile release of GnRH is required for production of LH and FSH. Pulses are released every 30–120 min. In men, there is a consistent frequency of pulses, but in women, the frequency varies depending on the phase of the menstrual cycle.[17] Several neuropeptides have been identified that exert a modulatory influence on GnRH secretion. Kisspeptin, which affects GnRH release, is widely acknowledged to be the initial trigger involved in the initiation of puberty. Neurokinin B and dynorphin are involved in the regulation of kisspeptin, and collectively, these three neuropeptides are known as KNDy neurons.[19]

GnRHas differ from native GnRH due to a chemical amino acid substitution at positions 6 and 10 in the GnRH molecule. This molecular change increases affinity for the GnRH receptor and decreases clearance by enzymatic removal.[20] When GnRH is present at a sustained continuous concentration, desensitization of the GnRH receptor occurs. It appears that multiple mechanisms may play a role in desensitization, one of which includes decreased mobilization of intracellular calcium. This occurs secondary to sustained stimulation

at the receptor by GnRH,[17] which in turn is thought to inhibit the release of LH.[8] Another important mechanism is related to an alteration in the levels of LH alpha and beta subunits in the presence of continuous GnRH exposure. While alpha subunit levels increase, the biologically active beta subunit levels decrease.[17] When used therapeutically, gonadal suppression is entirely reversed upon removal of GnRHa treatment.[18]

USE IN CENTRAL PRECOCIOUS PUBERTY

By far, the greatest source of knowledge regarding the clinical use of GnRHas in the pediatric population comes from experience with its use in CPP. When puberty develops prior to the onset of norms for racial background and ethnicity, it is considered precocious.[19] Specifically, CPP involves premature activation of the HPG axis[21] and has traditionally been defined as puberty starting before the age of 8 years in girls and before the age of 9 years in boys.[19] In addition to the age criteria, assessment for rapid progression, linear growth acceleration, and advancement of bone age are important aspects of the evaluation.[12,19] Many girls with idiopathic CPP will have a gradual progression of puberty with no compromise in final adult height. The major rationale for treatment is preservation of adult height potential, as there is a lack of evidence to support using GnRHas to delay menarche or ameliorate psychological outcomes. Girls younger than 6 years and boys younger than 9 years with rapidly progressive puberty have the greatest improvements in final height as a result of GnRHa treatment.[12]

Since the mid-1980s, long-acting GnRHas have been the standard of care for the treatment of CPP worldwide.[22] They have been shown to be effective and safe. Rapid-acting intranasal and subcutaneous forms are

TABLE 4.1				
Gonadotropin-Releasing Hormone Analogs				
(Limited to United States Formulations)	**Brand Name**	**Formulation**	**Dosage**	**Route**
Leuprolide	Lupron	Monthly	0.2–0.3 mg/kg per month	Intramuscular injection
		3-monthly	11.25 mg or 30 mg every 3 months	Intramuscular injection
Triptorelin	Triptodur	6-monthly	22.5 mg every 6 months	Intramuscular injection
Histrelin	Supprelin	Yearly[a]	50 mg every 12–24 months[a]	Subcutaneous implant
Nafarelin	Synarel	Twice daily	800 μg twice daily (starting dose)	Nasal spray

[a]Can be left in place for 2 years.

available, but depot formulations are recommended as compliance is improved with this method.[12] Monthly depot intramuscular injections are typically given at a dose of 0.2–0.3 mg/kg per month.[9,19] However, 3-monthly and 6-monthly forms are also now available.[12,13] An additional option for extended release is the histrelin subcutaneous implant which can be left in place for 2 years.[19,23] Table 4.1 summarizes formulations available in the United States.[12,13,24–27]

Initiation of GnRHa treatment results in cessation of pubertal progression, a return to a prepubertal growth velocity, and a decrease in the rate of skeletal maturation.[22] There is no evidence to support the need for routine laboratory monitoring while on treatment as long as clinical parameters indicate pubertal suppression. Response to treatment should be followed clinically with physical examination, assessment of growth, and intermittent determination of bone age.[12] Apparent clinical progression of puberty can indicate poor compliance, but treatment failure or the presence of an alternate diagnosis should be considered.[22]

GnRHas are extremely well tolerated, and most side effects are transient including rash, headaches, gastrointestinal issues, or hot flashes. Vaginal bleeding can occur after administration of the first dose in girls due to an initial flare in HPG axis activation with a concomitant increase in sex steroid levels prior to suppression.[22] Local reactions can occur in about 10–15% of cases and sterile abscesses have been reported. Anaphylaxis is very rare.[12]

The decision to stop treatment is individualized in each patient and incorporates consideration of the timing of normal puberty, individual height potential, psychological components, and patient and family preference. The average age of treatment cessation is 10.6–11.6 years.[12,22]

OUTCOMES IN CENTRAL PRECOCIOUS PUBERTY

Suppression of the HPG axis is reversible after discontinuation of a GnRHa, but variable information exists regarding long-term follow-up of treated patients.[26] Reproductive function in girls treated with GnRHas is not impaired. There are very limited data on outcomes in boys, but three small studies show intact reproductive function in them as well at the age of 15–18 years. While average time to menarche is approximately 16 months after stopping treatment, there is a wide variation of 2–61 months.[12] Time to menarche after treatment cessation appears to be inversely proportional to age,[26] whereas other factors such as bone age, breast Tanner stage, uterine development, or frequency of injections have not demonstrated uniformity with regard to affecting this interval of time.[20] The regularity of menstrual cycles in treated girls appears to be comparable to that observed in the normal adolescent population.[26] Although more data are needed to assess newer extended-release formulations, the mean time to menarche appears to be equivalent or slightly shorter on average in those treated with a histrelin implant compared with depot intramuscular GnRHas.[20,28] Fertility appears to be normal in women who were treated for CPP. In fact, GnRHa treatment appears to improve reproductive function in patients with a history of CPP, as those who are untreated require reproductive assistance more frequently.[20,29] Rates of pregnancy and live births do not appear to differ from those seen in the general population.[19]

The best height outcomes are achieved when treatment is initiated in girls who start treatment prior to the age of 6 years,[19,20] with height gains of 9–10 cm,[12] recognizing that height outcomes are variable among studies.[19] Evidence demonstrates that GnRHas are successful in halting further bone age advancement.[20] Girls treated between the age of 6 and 8 years show a moderate benefit in height outcome,[12] whereas those older than 8 years do not appear to benefit in terms of an increase in adult height.[19] There are insufficient data to allow for the establishment of analogous age cut-offs regarding height outcomes in boys.[12]

It is known that girls with CPP have higher rates of overweight and obesity prior to starting treatment with a GnRHa. This weight status continues throughout treatment and therefore does not appear to be secondary to the treatment itself. Body mass index does not increase further during GnRHa treatment.[19,26]

Although only a few studies are available, bone mineral density (BMD) does appear to decrease during GnRHa treatment, but once therapy is stopped, BMD returns to normal and ultimate accumulation of bone mass during adolescence is sufficient.[12,20,26]

There is controversy regarding an increased risk of polycystic ovarian syndrome (PCOS) in girls with CPP since studies suggest an increased incidence compared to unaffected individuals, but not necessarily attributed to the treatment itself.[19] There is a similar prevalence of PCOS in untreated patients with CPP which speaks against GnRHas as the cause.[26]

While it is known that girls with early puberty have earlier sexual risk-taking behaviors, it is unknown if this also applies to the CPP population and how GnRHas play into psychological outcomes.[12,19] While existing literature pertaining to psychosocial sequelae of early puberty in girls is inconsistent, studies have failed to find evidence of negative psychological consequences of CPP either at baseline or after 1 year.[30,31] Further studies are needed to investigate this topic.

There has been considerable interest in the potential use of GnRHas in children with normally timed puberty in whom the prognosis for adult height is deemed to be poor. This includes children with short stature, growth hormone deficiency, congenital adrenal hyperplasia, and profound primary hypothyroidism. Currently, there are insufficient data to support the use of GnRHas for any of these indications in routine clinical care, although more research is indisputably needed.[32]

USE IN GENDER-NONCONFORMING YOUTH

While awareness of gender dysphoria increased in the second half of the 20th century, recent years have witnessed an exponential rise in the number of referrals for gender-related concerns to pediatric endocrine and adolescent medicine clinics.[15] The World Professional Association for Transgender Health provides updated standard-of-care guidelines for the treatment of gender-nonconforming youth. Additionally, the Endocrine Society released updated clinical practice guidelines in 2017.[33] Both recommend GnRHas as the preferred method for pubertal suppression.[14,15]

Typically, the first stage of hormonal intervention consists of a puberty blocker to halt the progression of physical changes that are discordant with gender identity. It is not recommended to treat prepubertal children since intensification of gender dysphoria at the onset of puberty serves to reinforce the diagnosis. In addition, many children who are diagnosed in childhood ultimately desist and do not end up as transgender adults. Although a variety of strategies for suppressing endogenous sex steroids are available, GnRHas are the preferred approach. This allows the patient more time to reflect on their gender identity prior to embarking on the next phase of physical transition which consists of gender-affirming hormone (GAH) treatment which is considered only partially reversible.[14] When started in the early stages of puberty, GnRHas also prevent the development of secondary sexual characteristics, which often brings about an escalation in feelings of gender dysphoria, resulting in worse psychological outcomes in a population already at high-risk for psychopathologic comorbidities.[33] Some characteristics such as the Adam's apple, deeper voice, taller stature, male hair pattern, and body habitus in male-to-female (MTF) patients and breast development, female body habitus, and shorter stature in FTM patients are difficult or impossible to reverse once they have occurred. Thus, preventing these physical changes is associated with a more successful transition.[14,34] Another advantage of GnRHas is the fully reversible nature of this intervention. Once treatment is withdrawn, endogenous puberty concurrent with the patient's natal sex will resume and progress.[14,15]

Eligibility criteria for GnRHa treatment includes the presence of a long-lasting and intense pattern of gender dysphoria that worsens with the start of puberty, the absence of significant psychosocial or medical problems, sufficient medical capacity on the part of the patient and parent or guardian to give informed consent, and the presence of Tanner stage 2 or greater of pubertal development confirmed by a pediatric endocrinologist or other clinician.[14,15] Criteria for hormonal treatment also include confirmation of the diagnosis of gender dysphoria by a qualified mental health provider, and ongoing counseling during the period of transition is considered essential. Part of the informed consent process should involve the discussion of side effects and options for fertility preservation.[14] See Table 4.2 for a list of these eligibility criteria.[14,15]

When GnRHas are prescribed during the early stages of pubertal development, regression of existing physical changes often occurs, and any further progression is halted. For example, breast tissue and testicular size

> **TABLE 4.2**
> **Eligibility Criteria for Pubertal Suppression in Gender Nonconforming Youth**
>
> 1. The presence of a long-lasting and intense pattern of gender dysphoria that worsens with the start of puberty.
> 2. Psychosocial or medical problems that could interfere with treatment are addressed such that the adolescent is considered stable to start treatment.
> 3. The patient and parent or guardian has sufficient medical capacity to give informed consent. The discussion of side effects and options for fertility preservation should be involved.
> 4. The presence of Tanner stage 2 or greater of puberty confirmed by a pediatric endocrinologist or other clinician.
> 5. There are no medical contraindications to gonadotropin-releasing hormone analog treatment.

may decrease.[14] Monitoring during treatment includes anthropometric parameters (height, weight, Tanner staging) and laboratory assessments (LH, FSH, testosterone in MTF, estradiol in FTM) at baseline and every 6 months. Determination of bone age X-ray in patients with remaining growth potential and BMD assessed via dual-energy X-ray absorptiometry are recommended yearly.[14,34]

The age of initiation of GAH treatment varies, but typically occurs around the age of 16 years. The optimal length of time that a GnRHa should continue once GAH therapy has been initiated is unknown. As initial doses of testosterone or estrogen are not high enough to suppress gonadotropin production, it is important to continue the patient on a GnRHa at least during the early stages of GAH therapy. Current recommendations include continuing GnRHa treatment until gonadectomy. However, alternate options are available for patients in whom gonadectomy is not desired or prolonged treatment with a GnRHa is not feasible. Adult doses of testosterone may be sufficient monotherapy in FTM patients with the addition of a progestin if menstrual periods occur.[14,33] In MTF patients, an antiandrogen can be added to an estrogen regimen in lieu of a GnRHa.[14]

Although initiating GnRHa therapy early in puberty is considered optimal, many transgender youth do not seek medical intervention until well after endogenous puberty is essentially complete.[35] GnRHas are still considered appropriate in this setting as they represent the most potent means of rendering endogenous sex steroids to prepubertal values.

OPTIONS FOR TREATMENT

The exact same therapeutic armamentarium of GnRHa preparations are available for use in gender-variant patients as in those with CPP. One attractive option in addition to intramuscular formulations is the subcutaneous histrelin implant. The version marketed for children under the brand name Supprelin was approved by the FDA for use in CPP in 2007 and has been shown to be safe and effective.[36] This device is associated with favorable patient and parent satisfaction compared with depot intramuscular injections. The implant is generally well tolerated with the most common side effect, a local reaction at the implantation site, being temporary and self-limited. Retrieval of the device can be challenging due to a 22%–39% chance of breakage.[24] Despite this, fragments are easily retrievable through the original incision without the need for additional imaging or a different anesthetic technique.[36] The vast majority of implants can be placed and removed in the outpatient clinic under local anesthesia with child-life distraction and general anesthesia almost being never required.[24,36]

Another version of the histrelin implant that is marketed for adults is known by the brand name Vantas. Although only FDA approved for prostate cancer treatment in adult men,[37] it has been used successfully for pubertal suppression in transgender youth.[38] Both implants contain a total dose of 50 mg of histrelin acetate, but Supprelin releases 65 µg per day while Vantas releases 50 µg per day. Both are inserted subcutaneously into the upper arm, are FDA approved for 1 year, and decrease sex steroids to goal level by 1 month.[37,39] However, Supprelin contains enough medication to last for 2 years and provides effective suppression of the HPG axis for at least 24 months in children with CPP.[40]

OUTCOMES IN GENDER-NONCONFORMING YOUTH

The current landscape regarding outcomes of pubertal suppression in transgender youth is rife with large gaps in knowledge, and more long-term data regarding the safety of GnRHas in this setting are badly needed.[41] While much of what we know about these drugs can be inferred from their use in CPP, it is important to consider that their use in children with gender dysphoria occurs on an entirely different physiological and developmental background.[34] However, the limited evidence that is currently available suggests that when used appropriately in gender-variant patients, they are safe and effective at least in the short term.[33] Long-term effects are briefly reviewed here, with further discussion in subsequent chapters.

While gender dysphoria does not resolve completely with GnRHa therapy, its use has been associated with improved psychological functioning in areas of depression, anxiety, anger, overall functioning, and life satisfaction.[33,42] One argument against the use of GnRHas is that natal sex hormones are important for the development of gender identity and that adolescents may not possess the developmental foresight to understand the potential effects of pubertal suppression. However, the very real risk of increased psychological distress and concurrent rise in depression and suicidality caused by the development of secondary sexual characteristics that are inharmonious with gender identity is thought to outweigh this concern according to experts in the field.[43]

GnRHas result in adequate suppression of the HPG axis in transgender youth and can be used to manipulate adult height standard deviation score in patients in whom epiphyseal fusion has not yet occurred. Bone density z-scores appear to decrease significantly during pubertal suppression, but subsequently, bone accretion normalizes once GAH treatment is added. Studies are needed to assess long-term effects on bone health.[44] Changes in body composition include an increase in fat mass and a decrease in lean body mass during treatment.[14,33,44] It is unknown whether and in what way GnRHas may affect brain development.[44]

The first reported long-term follow-up of an FTM patient treated with a GnRHa and GAH with subsequent gender reassignment surgery was published in 2011 from the Netherlands. After 22 years of follow-up, this patient was doing well psychologically and had normal physical health, bone density, and body proportions. His final height was just below −2 standard deviations compared to natal males, and he wished to be taller. However, he had no regrets about his treatment process.[16] Similar findings were reported in a cohort of 55 young transgender adults who were evaluated approximately 7 years after completing transition and were found to have rates of well-being equivalent or better than their peers in the general population.[45]

Treatment with a GnRHa will suppress spermatogenesis and oocyte maturation. Suspending treatment for fertility preservation is an option but is complicated by the fact that gametogenesis occurs during the later stages of puberty, at which time substantial progression of secondary sexual characteristics has already occurred. The time to onset of gamete maturation after GnRHa cessation as well as the potential effects of prolonged GAH treatment on germ cell viability is currently unknown.[14] Surgical outcomes can also be impacted by GnRHa treatment in MTF patients who pursue creation of a neovagina, as sufficient phallic and scrotal skin may not be present. However, alternative surgical techniques using intestinal tissue have been successful.[33,46]

CHALLENGES IN CARE

Transgender youth may face many barriers to care including uninformed providers, long distance to centers providing transition services, lack of insurance approval for hormonal therapies, discrimination even within the medical environment, and/or lack of caregiver support and willingness to provide consent. Curriculum for the care of transgender patients in current medical education is lacking with only a few medical schools providing this type of instruction.[38,47] While GnRHas are the standard of care for pubertal suppression, the FDA has not approved their use for pubertal suppression for gender dysphoria, so current prescriptions are all considered "off label."[38]

Insurance denial for hormone treatment is a substantial barrier leading to large out-of-pocket expenses for families. The high costs of GnRHas make them out of reach for many. Compounding the burden is the large cost differential between GnRHa formulations that are marketed for pediatric versus adult use.[48] For example, the cost difference between the 3-monthly formulation of Lupron Depot ($4800) compared to the 3-monthly preparation of Lupron Depot-Ped ($9700) is approximately $4900. The cost of the pediatric subcutaneous histrelin implant (Supprelin) is approximately $35,000 compared with the adult subcutaneous histrelin implant (Vantas) which is approximately $4400, resulting in a difference of approximately $30,600.[49,50] The use of some mail order pharmacies or Vantas represents potential ways of limiting costs for families paying out of pocket for hormonal treatment.[38,48]

CONCLUSION

In conclusion, within the historical context of GnRHa use in the pediatric population, the employment of this class of medications in gender-variant children and adolescents represents a new frontier. While initial knowledge is reassuring, many important questions remain pertaining to both physical and psychological consequences of suppressing normally timed puberty, sometimes for upwards of 7 years, in these vulnerable patients. Long-term, carefully conducted prospective studies are needed to further delineate the risks and benefits of GnRHas in transgender youth.

REFERENCES

1. Fink G. 60 YEARS OF NEUROENDOCRINOLOGY: MEMOIR: Harris' neuroendocrine revolution: of portal vessels and self-priming. *J Endocrinol*. 2015;226(2):T13−T24.
2. Antunes JL, Muraszko K. The vascular supply of the hypothalamus-pituitary axis. *Acta Neurochir Suppl (Wien)*. 1990;47:42−47.
3. Jewelewicz R, Dyrenfurth I, Warren M, Wiele RV. Clinical studies with gonadotropin-releasing hormone. *Bull N Y Acad Med*. 1974;50(10):1097.
4. Schally A, Arimura A, Kastin A, et al. Gonadotropin-releasing hormone: one polypeptide regulates secretion of luteinizing and follicle-stimulating hormones. *Science*. 1971;173(4001):1036−1038.
5. Nobel Media AB. *Physiology or Medicine 1977-Press Release*. *Nobelprize.Org*; 2014. http://www.nobelprize.org/nobel_prizes/medicine/laureates/1977/press.html.
6. Andreyko JL, Marshall LA, Dumesic DA, Jaffe RB. Therapeutic uses of gonadotropin-releasing hormone analogs. *Obstet Gynecol Surv*. 1987;42(1):1−21.
7. Belchetz P, Plant T, Nakai Y, Keogh E, Knobil E. Hypophysial responses to continuous and intermittent delivery of hypopthalamic gonadotropin-releasing hormone. *Science*. 1978;202(4368):631−633.
8. Conn PD, Michael P, Crowley Jr M, William F. Gonadotropin-releasing hormone and its analogs. *Annu Rev Med*. 1994;45(1):391−405.
9. Breyer P, Haider A, Pescovitz OH. Gonadotropin-releasing hormone agonists in the treatment of girls with central precocious puberty. *Clin Obstet Gynecol*. 1993;36(3):764−772.
10. Abbott Laboratories Takeda Pharmaceutical Company Limited. *Highlights of Prescribing Information Lupron Depotped*; 2011. https://www.accessdata.fda.gov/drugsatfda_docs/label/2011/020263s036lbl.pdf.
11. Neely E, Hintz R, Parker B, et al. Two-year results of treatment with depot leuprolide acetate for central precocious puberty. *J Pediatr*. 1992;121(4):634−640.
12. Carel J-C, Eugster EA, Rogol A, Ghizzoni L, Palmert MR. Consensus statement on the use of gonadotropin-releasing hormone analogs in children. *Pediatrics*. 2009;123(4):e752−e762.
13. Klein K, Yang J, Aisenberg J, et al. Efficacy and safety of triptorelin 6-month formulation in patients with central precocious puberty. *J Pediatr Endocrinol Metab*. 2016;29(11):1241−1248.
14. Hembree WC, Cohen-Kettenis PT, Gooren L, et al. Endocrine treatment of gender-dysphoric/gender-incongruent persons: an endocrine society clinical practice guideline. *J Clin Endocrinol Metab*. 2017;102.
15. World Professional Association for Transgender Health. *Standards of Care for the Health of Transsexual, Transgender, and Gender Nonconforming People 7th Version*; 2011. http://www.wpath.org/site_page.cfm?pk_association_webpage_menu=1351.
16. Cohen-Kettenis PT, Schagen SE, Steensma TD, de Vries AL, Delemarre-van de Waal HA. Puberty suppression in a gender-dysphoric adolescent: a 22-year follow-up. *Arch Sex Behav*. 2011;40(4):843−847.
17. Millar RP, Newton CL. Current and future applications of GnRH, kisspeptin and neurokinin B analogues. *Nat Rev Endocrinol*. 2013;9(8):451−466.
18. Heger S, Sippell WG, Partsch C-J. Gonadotropin-releasing hormone analogue treatment for precocious puberty. *Abnorm Puberty*. 2005;8:94−125.
19. Fuqua JS. Treatment and outcomes of precocious puberty: an update. *J Clin Endocrinol Metab*. 2013;98(6):2198−2207.
20. Guaraldi F, Beccuti G, Gori D, Ghizzoni L. Management of endocrine disease: long-term outcomes of the treatment of central precocious puberty. *Eur J Endocrinol*. 2016;174(3):R79−R87.
21. Mul D, Hughes I. The use of GnRH agonists in precocious puberty. *Eur J Endocrinol*. 2008;159(suppl 1):S3−S8.
22. Latronico AC, Brito VN, Carel J-C. Causes, diagnosis, and treatment of central precocious puberty. *Lancet Diabetes Endocrinol*. 2016;4(3):265−274.
23. Chen M, Eugster EA. Central precocious puberty: update on diagnosis and treatment. *Pediatr Drugs*. 2015;17(4):273−281.
24. Eugster EA. Experience with the histrelin implant in pediatric patients. *Adv Ther Pediatr Endocrinol Diabetol*. 2016;30:54−59.
25. Carel J-C, Leger J. Precocious puberty. *N Engl J Med*. 2008;358(22):2366−2377.
26. Thornton P, Silverman LA, Geffner ME, Neely EK, Gould E, Danoff TM. Review of outcomes after cessation of gonadotropin-releasing hormone agonist treatment of girls with precocious puberty. *Pediatr Endocrinol Rev*. 2014;11(3):306−317.
27. Bertelloni S, Baroncelli GI. Current pharmacotherapy of central precocious puberty by GnRH analogs: certainties and uncertainties. *Expert Opin Pharmacother*. 2013;14(12):1627−1639.
28. Fisher MM, Lemay D, Eugster EA. Resumption of puberty in girls and boys following removal of the histrelin implant. *J Pediatr*. 2014;164(4):912−916.e911.
29. Lazar L, Meyerovitch J, Vries L, Phillip M, Lebenthal Y. Treated and untreated women with idiopathic precocious puberty: long-term follow-up and reproductive outcome between the third and fifth decades. *Clin Endocrinol*. 2014;80(4):570−576.
30. Schoelwer MJ, Donahue KL, Bryk K, Didrick P, Berenbaum SA, Eugster EA. Psychological assessment of mothers and their daughters at the time of diagnosis of precocious puberty. *Int J Pediatr Endocrinol*. 2015;2015(1):5.

31. Schoelwer MJ, Donahue KL, Didrick P, Eugster EA. One-year follow-up of girls with precocious puberty and their mothers: do psychological assessments change over time or with treatment? *Horm Res Paediatr.* 2017; 88(5).

32. Eugster EA. The use of gonadotropin-releasing hormone analogs beyond precocious puberty. *J Pediatr.* 2015; 167(2):481−485.

33. Mahfouda S, Moore JK, Siafarikas A, Zepf FD, Lin A. Puberty suppression in transgender children and adolescents. *Lancet Diabetes Endocrinol.* 2017;5.

34. Vance SR, Ehrensaft D, Rosenthal SM. Psychological and medical care of gender nonconforming youth. *Pediatrics.* 2014;134(6):1184−1192.

35. Chen M, Fuqua J, Eugster EA. Characteristics of referrals for gender dysphoria over a 13-year period. *J Adolesc Health.* 2016;58(3):369−371.

36. Davis JS, Alkhoury F, Burnweit C. Surgical and anesthetic considerations in histrelin capsule implantation for the treatment of precocious puberty. *J Pediatr Surg.* 2014; 49(5):807−810.

37. Endo Pharmaceuticals Solutions Inc. Vantas Package Insert. 2017. http://www.endo.com/File%20Library/Products /Prescribing%20Information/Vantas_prescribing_information. html.

38. Shumer DE, Nokoff NJ, Spack NP. Advances in the care of transgender children and adolescents. *Adv Pediatr.* 2016; 63(1):79−102.

39. Indevus Pharmaceuticals. *Supprelin LA: Highlights of Prescribing Information;* 2007. https://www.accessdata.fda. gov/drugsatfda_docs/label/2008/022058s003lbl.pdf.

40. Lewis KA, Goldyn AK, West KW, Eugster EA. A single histrelin implant is effective for 2 years for treatment of central precocious puberty. *J Pediatr.* 2013;163(4): 1214−1216.

41. Olson-Kennedy J, Cohen-Kettenis PT, Kreukels BP, et al. Research priorities for gender nonconforming/transgender youth: gender identity development and biopsychosocial outcomes. *Curr Opin Endocrinol Diabetes Obes.* 2016; 23(2):172−179.

42. De Vries AL, Steensma TD, Doreleijers TA, Cohen-Kettenis PT. Puberty suppression in adolescents with gender identity disorder: a prospective follow-up study. *J Sex Med.* 2011;8(8):2276−2283.

43. Leibowitz SF, Telingator C. Assessing gender identity concerns in children and adolescents: evaluation, treatments, and outcomes. *Curr Psychiatry Rep.* 2012;14(2):111−120.

44. Delemarre-van de Waal HA, Cohen-Kettenis PT. Clinical management of gender identity disorder in adolescents: a protocol on psychological and paediatric endocrinology aspects. *Eur J Endocrinol.* 2006;155(suppl 1): S131−S137.

45. De Vries AL, McGuire JK, Steensma TD, Wagenaar EC, Doreleijers TA, Cohen-Kettenis PT. Young adult psychological outcome after puberty suppression and gender reassignment. *Pediatrics.* 2014;134(4):696−704.

46. Colebunders B, Brondeel S, D'Arpa S, Hoebeke P, Monstrey S. An update on the surgical treatment for transgender patients. *Sex Med Rev.* 2017;5(1):103−109.

47. Radix A, Silva M. Beyond the guidelines: challenges, controversies, and unanswered questions. *Pediatr Ann.* 2014; 43(6):e145−e150.

48. Stevens J, Gomez-Lobo V, Pine-Twaddell E. Insurance coverage of puberty blocker therapies for transgender youth. *Pediatrics.* 2015;136(6):1029−1031.

49. Red Book Online. Histrelin; 2018. https://pediatriccare. solutions.aap.org/drug.aspx?gbosid=171001.

50. Red Book Online. Leuprolide; 2018. https://pediatriccare. solutions.aap.org/drug.aspx?gbosid=171217#sec_ 180307445.

CHAPTER 5

Rationale for the Initiation, Use, and Monitoring of GnRHa in Gender Non-conforming Youth

JEREMI M. CARSWELL, MD • STEPHANIE A. ROBERTS, MD

INTRODUCTION

Gonadotropin-releasing hormone (GnRH) agonists, commonly referred to as puberty-blocking agents, while most commonly thought of as a treatment for prevention of secondary sexual characteristics, have psychosocial benefits that span the transition process. They may also provide relief even for the older adolescent. They allow the adolescent to continue to explore their gender identity without the burden of unwanted physical development. As a cornerstone of modern adolescent transgender care, it is critical to recognize the profound positive impact this intervention can have on not only the patient but also their family unit, their providers, and their interaction with their greater social world. The use of GnRH agonists is a safe, effective, and, most importantly, reversible intervention whose benefits outweigh harm in appropriately selected patients.

RATIONALE

When a child or adolescent presents to a gender program with a desire for transition but is not yet at the age of majority for gender-affirming hormones, the use of GnRH agonist affords the time to explore their gender identity. The most accessible and visible benefit is physical, encompassing a wide range of attributes including facial structure, height, musculature, and body shape. In a prepubertal state, these are quite similar between boys and girls. This accounts for the prepubertal child to pass easily in their affirmed gender. Once exposed to sex steroids, however, these features may become exceptionally identifying to the assigned gender. The face is probably the most distressing, as it is so easily "gendered" and yet unable to be covered or modified without surgery. Studies on facial

recognition demonstrate rapid and exceptionally accurate identification of a face as male or female.[1−3]

Other undesired secondary sexual characteristics cause dysphoria in adolescents and may be preventable with the use of a GnRH agonist or "blocker." In the transmasculine patient, prevention of breast growth will avoid breast dysphoria and chest reconstructive surgery. Similarly, in our experience, many transmasculine teens that have transitioned postpubertally are very dismayed about their hip shape and express their desire to have a more masculine shape with narrower hips. In the transfeminine patient, the effects of testosterone are powerful and permanent including angularity of the face, a deep voice, and prominent cricothyroid cartilage, or Adam's apple.

From a medical standpoint, the use of GnRH agonist also allows for lower doses of gender-affirming hormones if that becomes part of a youth's medical transition in the future (Fig. 5.1).

The mental health benefits of using these agents were first studied by the transgender clinic in the Netherlands in the first group of children to use GnRH agonists in a systematic way.[4] They analyzed measures of psychosocial well-being at first assessment and then just prior to the initiation of gender-affirming hormones. They found a significant decrease in behavioral and emotional problems, fewer reported depressive symptoms but stable feelings of anxiety and anger, and an improvement in general function. Importantly, there was no reduction in gender dysphoria until after the time of gender-affirming surgery. It should be noted that these patients had a mean age of just over 14 years for assigned males and 15 years for assigned females, most of whom had full breast development and menarche and thus did not actually experience the full potential benefit of this

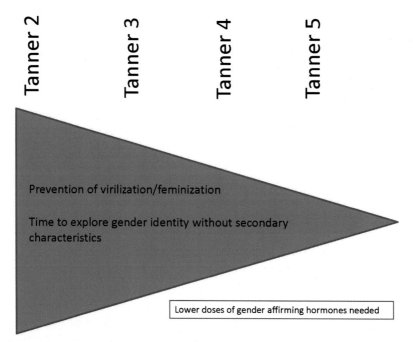

FIG. 5.1 Schematic representation of the use of GnRH agonist that permits lower doses of gender-affirming hormones. There is greatest physical benefit at tanner 2 that tapers as an individual matures.

intervention, suggesting outcomes could have been potentially even better with earlier implementation.

When adolescents present later in puberty, pubertal blockade is a consideration for prevention of late effects of gonadal steroids, particularly in assigned males who may not yet have thick facial hair or a broad chest. Compared to other agents commonly used for the purpose of testosterone suppression, including progestagens and spironolactone, GnRH agonist typically suppress testosterone so effectively that they allow for the use of physiologic doses of estrogen replacement compared to supraphysiologic doses of estrogen, which are typically administered in older treatment protocols for adults.[5]

INITIATION

Initiation of GnRH agonist is recommended by current guidelines in the early stages of puberty.[5] This is based on prior studies showing that a large percentage of gender dysphoric youth did not maintain their transgender identity as adults and instead affirmed a homosexual sexual orientation and cisgendered gender identity.[6] Approximately a dozen studies have been published on this topic, dating back to the 1960s. However, these studies are controversial within the scientific and transgender community due to small sample size and design flaws, including limitations of their retrospective nature such as recall bias. One of the largest studies from these, performed in the Netherlands, showed that the extremeness of gender insistence in childhood was one predictor of persistence of a transgender gender identity as an adult,[7] but this finding has not been replicated in a large series. Medical transition (e.g., implementing GnRH agonist therapy to prevent puberty before it begins) is not recommended for prepubertal youth, as the available evidence suggests that experiencing some amount of pubertal development is important for gender identity development.[5] As this field and the diagnostic criteria for establishing the diagnosis of gender dysphoria have changed, so may our understanding factors associated with persistence and desistance of transgender and gender nonconforming identities.

Early pubertal onset, which is the recommended time for initiation of GnRH agonist, can be assessed by Tanner staging, a scale commonly used to assess breast development in assigned girls and genital growth in assigned boys[8] (Fig. 5.2). A scale for pubic hair

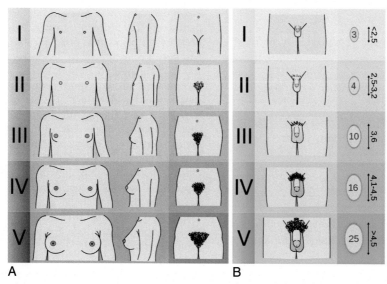

FIG. 5.2 **(A)** Tanner staging for breast and public hair (female). **(B)** Tanner staging for breast and pubic hair (male). ((A) Adapted from https://commons.wikimedia.org/wiki/File%3ATanner_scale-female.svg By M·Komorniczak -talk-, polish wikipedist. (B) Adapted from https://commons.wikimedia.org/wiki/File% 3ATanner_scale-male.svg By M·Komorniczak -talk-, polish wikipedist.)

development exists for both assigned girls and boys. Five stages exist for each scale with Tanner stage I for prepubertal children increasing to Tanner stage V of mature adult development.[8] In assigned girls, the hallmark of pubertal onset is breast budding with concomitant increase in growth velocity leading to the pubertal growth spurt. In assigned boys, the first stage is enlargement of testicular volume with the pubertal growth spurt in the later stages of puberty compared to assigned females and thus is not likely to be seen in early puberty development in assigned males.[9]

The onset of puberty should be confirmed by these physical exam findings by an experienced clinician as isolated adrenarche can sometimes be confused for the onset of true central puberty.[10] The appearance of adult body odor, axillary hair, and pubic hair may be due to normal age-related activation of the adrenal gland or adrenarche. This commonly co-occurs with central puberty but may occur independently.[11]

GnRH agonist therapy can be implemented as early as Tanner stage II–III breast or genital staging.

The use of a GnRH agonist may also be considered in mid-puberty or in the postpubertal period to prevent further pubertal progression in the former, or effectively inhibit unwanted natal sex steroid production in the latter. This includes uterine bleeding in mid to late pubertal assigned females.[12] The youth and family should be counseled that most secondary sexual characteristics that have already developed will not likely regress unless treatment is initiated in the very early stages. Additionally, in transgender and nonbinary youth who may not desire gender-affirming hormones, providers may be asked to provide GnRH agonist to achieve a prolonged agonadal state. These patients and families should be counseled about the potential risks such as the effect of estrogen deprivation on bony mineralization, which may not fully recover.[13,14] Focusing therapy to relieve particularly dysphoric issues, such as the use of a progestin for unwanted menstrual bleeding or top surgery for unwanted female breasts may be preferred modes of medical transition in those without desire to eventually move forward with gender-affirming hormones.[12] This is an area with any evidence or expert opinion guidelines to guide clinical practice and is a new era of medical transition.

MONITORING

Monitoring of an adolescent while on pubertal suppression is multifaceted, involving clinical, hormonal, and radiographic modalities and should be performed by an experienced clinician. It is important to follow not only efficacy of GnRH agonist therapy but also potential adverse effects, such as decreasing linear growth and

TABLE 5.1
Baseline and Follow-Up Protocol During Suppression of Puberty

EVERY 3–6 MONTHS
Anthropometry: height, weight, sitting height, blood pressure, Tanner stages
EVERY 6–12 MONTHS
Laboratory: LH, FSH, E2/T, 25-hydroxy vitamin D
EVERY 1–2 YEARS
Bone density using DXA
Bone age on X-ray of the left hand (if clinically indicated)

Adapted from Hembree et al. (5).
DXA, dual-energy X-ray absorptiometry; *E2*, estradiol; *FSH*, follicle stimulating hormone; *LH*, luteinizing hormone; *T*, testosterone.

bone density. Monitoring will vary based on the type of GnRH agonist implement.

The frequency for monitoring adolescents under pubertal suppression is shown as recommended by current guidelines (Table 5.1); however, clinical judgment may allow for less intense surveillance.

Clinical Monitoring

Baseline monitoring should include assessment of weight, height, and blood pressure and reassessment of arthrometric parameters at regular intervals once on GnRH agonist therapy.[5] Tanner staging of pubic hair and of breasts in assigned females and genitalia in assigned males should be reassessed at each visit. Clinically, treatment success is defined by prevention of secondary sex characteristics and a prepubertal growth velocity. Youth should be counseled that secondary sexual characteristics may initially advance, including the potential of vaginal bleeding in an assigned female, before suppression of the hypothalamic–gonadal axis occurs.[15] Conversely, GnRH agonist failure would be suggested by progression in breast development and a pubertal growth velocity in assigned females and testicular growth in assigned males. It is important to note adrenal hormones, such as dehydroepiandrosterone sulfate, dehydroepiandrosterone, and androstenedione, are unaffected by the suppression of the hypothalamic–pituitary–gonadal axis with GnRH agonist therapy, therefore there will likely be progression of pubic and axillary hair, and persistence (or development) of apocrine odor and acne.[11]

Families should be counseled that while on GnRH agonist therapy, growth velocity will remain at a prepubertal growth rate (and in fact there may be a period of "catch-down" growth, when the velocity decreases to below that of a typical prepubertal child) and youth may appear to decelerate on their growth curves compared to pubertal peers. This is because the pubertal growth spurt is in part fueled by sex steroids, and withdrawal or prevention of these sex steroids is associated with a growth rate that more closely approximates that of a prepubertal child, approximately 4–7 cm/year.[16] This can appear alarming when charted on the growth curve, as it may appear that the adolescent has growth failure but is in fact expected. One study suggests low-dose estrogen may be used to optimize linear growth during treatment with GnRH agonist if the growth velocity falls below a normal prepubertal child, however it not the standard of care.[17]

An increased body mass index, due to increased fat mass, has been observed in the GnRH-treated precocious and early puberty population.[18,19] When examined closely, however, some studies note an inverse relationship with pretreatment weight and weight gain.[20,21] That is, the most significant weight gain was in previously normal weight patients, whereas baseline obese children did not experience this increase. Other studies have not found this association.[22–25] To our knowledge there are no published data regarding weight gain and the use of GnRHa in the gender nonconforming population, for whom blockade typically occurs at later ages. It is recommended, however, to monitor weight (and consequently body mass index) at regular intervals and provide lifestyle counseling as indicated.

Hormone Monitoring

Serum gonadotropins [luteinizing hormone (LH) and follicle stimulating hormone (FSH)], and estradiol or testosterone levels are typically assessed to confirm pubertal onset. In the early stages of pubertal development, gonadotropins are best obtained in the early morning, as they may be falsely low later in the day due to circadian pattern of gonadotropin secretion in the early stages of puberty.[26] Stimulation testing using leuprolide can be performed if laboratory testing is equivocal but is not typically required.[27]

It should be noted that much of the knowledge on biochemical monitoring is adapted from the literature on precocious puberty. The "gold-standard" for assessing adequacy of therapy is measurement of LH after luteinizing hormone-releasing hormone (LHRH) stimulation,[28] which is no longer available in the United States. A consensus statement on the use of

GnRH agonist in children published in 2009 did not recommend routine testing of random or stimulated measurement of gonadotropins (LH, FSH) or sex steroids[29] but did note that an elevated unstimulated LH level could indicate lack of suppression. This, however, has been challenged by authors who noted that random LH levels often remain in the pubertal range during histrelin therapy.[30–32] In one prospective study looking at children with precocious puberty, there was a 59% prevalence of LH > 0.03 IU/L (the accepted pubertal value), despite none of the children having GnRHa-stimulated LH levels that exceeded the cutoff for pubertal LH value and there being no evidence of clinical progression.[30] Other studies have replicated these findings with leuprolide depot.[33,34]

Estrogen and testosterone levels (for assigned females and males, respectively) should be followed and are likely more reliable for detecting treatment failure. In one early study looking at the efficacy of histrelin implant in children with central precocious puberty, the mean estradiol levels measured by radioimmunoassay were 5.9 ± 2.37 pg/mL (compared to 24.5 ± 22.27 pg/mL at pretreatment). (**4U**). A later study by the same group again showed that estradiol levels remain suppressed, even when using the more sensitive liquid chromatography—tandem mass spectrometry.[35] This may not be as reliable in patients on leuprolide, however. One study found a 23% rate of elevated estradiol in LHRH-stimulated proven suppressed patients on leuprolide,[36] while previous studies have demonstrated an overlap of estradiol levels in prepubertal and pubertal girls.[28,37,38] Testosterone levels have been shown to remain suppressed during treatment with Lupron injections and in studies using the histrelin implant.[35,39]

If stimulated LH levels are desired to monitor GnRH efficacy, the timing of the blood draw will vary based on the method of GnRH administration. For example, with monthly intramuscular leuprolide injections, a LH level drawn 30—60 min after the first or second injections can be assessed with a stimulated LH level <3 mIU/mL consistent with pubertal suppression.[40] For a subcutaneous histrelin implant, unstimulated gonadotropin and sex steroid levels can be drawn any time after the first month of treatment and are not expected to be suppressed to prepubertal levels.[30,35]

Current Endocrine Society Guidelines[5] do recommend obtaining both LH and FSH levels every 6—12 months, with the recognition that there is insufficient evidence for a specific short-term monitoring scheme and will vary based on preparation of GnRH agonist. In assigned girls, serum LH may be sufficient to follow for monitoring, especially given limitations of most estradiol assays. In assigned boys, the total testosterone level alone may be sufficient as evidence of ongoing pubertal suppression. The lack of progression of secondary sexual characteristics and assessment of growth velocity in the prepubertal range (4—6 cm/year)[41] are important adjuncts to biochemical monitoring.

Radiographic Monitoring

At baseline, a bone age X-ray, a radiograph of the left hand and wrist, and dual-energy X-ray absorptiometry (DXA) scan are recommended.[5] Bone age X-rays can be repeated every 1—2 years to follow skeletal maturity, which is expected to advance more slowly in youth under pubertal suppression compared to cisgendered peers. The use of bone age to predict a final adult height is typically performed by endocrinologists; however, there are no current standards to predict which gender should be used for height predictions in the setting of gender-affirming hormones. Nonetheless, approximation of adult height may influence the ultimate timing and tempo of gender-affirming hormones if desired by the transgender youth as part of medical transition to help optimize or attenuate final adult height.

Additionally, a bone health history, including any history of fracture, as well as calcium and vitamin D intake should be assessed, and youth should be counseled on modifiable risk factors to optimize bone health [Endocrine Society]. The 25-hydroxy vitamin D levels should be assessed in all patients and treated with vitamin D replacement if found to be insufficient or deficient. The cutoff for a normal vitamin D level is controversial; however, most endocrinologists endorse treating a vitamin 25-hydroxy vitamin D level below 20 ng/mL, with a goal to raise the serum level above 30 ng/mL.[42] Baseline DXA scan should be assessed and interpreted within standards for the assigned gender. DXA scans must be interpreted against *bone-age*-matched control standards and reported as z-scores, not T-scores which are comparisons to the density of a healthy young adult. Bone density parameters (e.g., z-scores) should be adjusted for bone age, a marker of skeletal maturity, and extreme tall or short stature, both of which can influence testing results.[43] In severe cases, low bone density may lead to consider gender-affirming hormones earlier or consideration of a low dose of estradiol for bone health protection.

CONCLUSION

The use of GnRH agonist in gender dysphoric youth is a reversible option that can be initiated in the early stages of puberty or even in the mid- or postpubertal stages of development. Monitoring of laboratory and radiologic parameters should be performed by a transcompetent medical provider. Prolonged use of GnRH agonist in transgender and nonbinary youth to allow individuals to remain in an agonadal state, without any desire for gender-affirming hormones, should be exercised with caution. Additional long-term outcome studies looking at benefits and risks of transgender youth treated with GnRH agonist are needed to best care for this special population.

REFERENCES

1. Gross CG. Processing the facial image: a brief history. Am Psychol. 2005;60. https://doi.org/10.1037/0003-066X.60.8.755.
2. Walker M, Wänke M. Caring or daring? Exploring the impact of facial masculinity/femininity and gender category information on first impressions. PLoS One. 2017;12. https://doi.org/10.1371/journal.pone.0181306.
3. O'Toole AJ, Deffenbacher KA, Valentin D, McKee K, Huff D, Abdi H. The perception of face gender: the role of stimulus structure in recognition and classification. Mem Cognit. 1998;26. https://doi.org/10.3758/BF03211378.
4. de Vries ALC, Steensma TD, Doreleijers TAH, Cohen-Kettenis PT. Puberty suppression in adolescents with gender identity disorder: a prospective follow-up study. J Sex Med. 2011;8(8):2276–2283. https://doi.org/10.1111/j.1743-6109.2010.01943.x.
5. Hembree WC, Cohen-Kettenis PT, Gooren L, et al. Endocrine Treatment of Gender-Dysphoric/Gender-Incongruent Persons: an Endocrine Society* Clinical Practice Guideline. J Clin Endocrinol Metab. 2017;102:3869–3903. https://doi.org/10.1210/jc.2017-01658.
6. Wallien MS, Cohen-Kettenis PT. Psychosexual outcome of gender-dysphoric children. J Am Acad Child Adolesc Psychiatry. 2008;47(12):1413–1423. https://doi.org/10.1097/CHI.0b013e31818956b9.
7. Steensma TD, McGuire JK, Kreukels BPC, Beekman AJ, Cohen-Kettenis PT. Factors associated with desistence and persistence of childhood gender dysphoria: a quantitative follow-up study. J Am Acad Child Adolesc Psychiatry. 2013;52(6):582–590. https://doi.org/10.1016/j.jaac.2013.03.016.
8. Tanner JM. Growth at Adolescence. Springfield, IL: Thomas; 1962.
9. Bordini B, Rosenfield RL. Normal pubertal development: Part II: clinical aspects of puberty. Pediatr Rev. 2011; 32(7):281–292. https://doi.org/10.1542/pir.32-7-281.
10. Kaplowitz P, Bloch C. Section on Endocrinology, American Academy of pediatrics. Evaluation and referral of children with signs of early puberty. Pediatrics. 2016;137(1): e20153732. https://doi.org/10.1542/peds.2015-3732.
11. Pinyerd B, Zipf WB. Puberty—timing is everything!. J Pediatr Nurs. 2005;20(2):75–82. https://doi.org/10.1016/j.pedn.2004.12.011.
12. Carswell JM, Roberts SA. Induction and maintenance of Amenorrhea in transmasculine and nonbinary adolescents. Transgend Health. 2017;2(1):195–201. https://doi.org/10.1089/trgh.2017.0021.
13. Klink D, Caris M, Heijboer A, van Trotsenburg M, Rotteveel J. Bone mass in young adulthood following gonadotropin-releasing hormone analog treatment and cross-sex hormone treatment in adolescents with gender dysphoria. J Clin Endocrinol Metab. 2015;100(2): E270–E275. https://doi.org/10.1210/jc.2014-2439.
14. Vlot MC, Klink DT, den Heijer M, Blankenstein MA, Rotteveel J, Heijboer AC. Effect of pubertal suppression and cross-sex hormone therapy on bone turnover markers and bone mineral apparent density (BMAD) in transgender adolescents. Bone. 2017;95:11–19. https://doi.org/10.1016/j.bone.2016.11.008.
15. Lahlou N, Carel JC, Chaussain JL, Roger M. Pharmacokinetics and pharmacodynamics of GnRH agonists: clinical implications in pediatrics. J Pediatr Endocrinol Metab. 2000;13(suppl 1):723–737. http://www.ncbi.nlm.nih.gov/pubmed/10969915.
16. Tanner JM, Davies PS. Clinical longitudinal standards for height and height velocity for North American children. J Pediatr. 1985;107(3):317–329. http://www.ncbi.nlm.nih.gov/pubmed/3875704.
17. Lampit M, Golander A, Guttmann H, Hochberg Z. Estrogen mini-dose replacement during GnRH agonist therapy in central precocious puberty: a pilot study. J Clin Endocrinol Metab. 2002;87(2):687–690. https://doi.org/10.1210/jcem.87.2.8242.
18. Taşcilar ME, Bilir P, Akinci A, et al. The effect of gonadotropin-releasing hormone analog treatment (leuprolide) on body fat distribution in idiopathic central precocious puberty. Turk J Pediatr. 2011;53(1):27–33. http://www.ncbi.nlm.nih.gov/pubmed/21534336.
19. Chiumello G, Brambilla P, Guarneri MP, Russo G, Manzoni P, Sgaramella P. Precocious puberty and body composition: effects of GnRH analog treatment. J Pediatr Endocrinol Metab. 2000;13(suppl 1):791–794. http://www.ncbi.nlm.nih.gov/pubmed/10969923.
20. Kim SW, Kim YB, Lee JE, et al. The influence of gonadotropin releasing hormone agonist treatment on the body weight and body mass index in girls with idiopathic precocious puberty and early puberty. Ann Pediatr Endocrinol Metab. 2017;22(2):95. https://doi.org/10.6065/apem.2017.22.2.95.
21. Arcari AJ, Gryngarten MG, Freire AV, et al. Body mass index in girls with idiopathic central precocious puberty during and after treatment with GnRH analogues. Int J Pediatr Endocrinol. 2016;2016(1):15. https://doi.org/10.1186/s13633-016-0033-7.
22. Głab E, Barg E, Wikiera B, Grabowski M, Noczyńska A. Influence of GnRH analog therapy on body mass in central precocious puberty. Pediatr Endocrinol Diabetes Metab. 2009;15(1):7–11. http://www.ncbi.nlm.nih.gov/pubmed/19454183.

23. Heger S, Partsch C-J, Sippell WG. Long-term outcome after depot gonadotropin-releasing hormone agonist treatment of central precocious puberty: final height, body proportions, body composition, bone mineral density, and reproductive function. *J Clin Endocrinol Metab.* 1999;84(12): 4583−4590. https://doi.org/10.1210/jcem.84.12.6203.

24. Palmert MR, Mansfield MJ, Crowley WF, Crigler JF, Crawford JD, Boepple PA. Is obesity an outcome of gonadotropin-releasing hormone agonist administration? Analysis of growth and body composition in 110 patients with central precocious puberty. *J Clin Endocrinol Metab.* 1999;84(12):4480−4488. https://doi.org/10.1210/jcem. 84.12.6204.

25. Shiasi Arani K, Heidari F. Gonadotropin-releasing hormone agonist therapy and obesity in girls. *Int J Endocrinol Metab.* 2015;13(3). https://doi.org/10.5812/ijem.23085v2.

26. Jakacki RI, Kelch RP, Sauder SE, Lloyd JS, Hopwood NJ, Marshall JC. Pulsatile secretion of luteinizing hormone in children. *J Clin Endocrinol Metab.* 1982;55(3): 453−458. https://doi.org/10.1210/jcem-55-3-453.

27. Sathasivam A, Garibaldi L, Shapiro S, Godbold J, Rapaport R. Leuprolide stimulation testing for the evaluation of early female sexual maturation. *Clin Endocrinol (Oxf).* 2010;73(3):375−381. https://doi.org/10.1111/j.1365-2265.2010.03796.x.

28. Lee PA. Laboratory monitoring of children with precocious puberty. *Arch Pediatr Adolesc Med.* 1994;148(4):369−376. http://www.ncbi.nlm.nih.gov/pubmed/8148936.

29. Carel J-C, Eugster EA, Rogol A, et al. Consensus statement on the use of gonadotropin-releasing hormone analogs in children. *Pediatrics.* 2009;123(4):e752−e762. https://doi.org/10.1542/peds.2008-1783.

30. Neely EK, Silverman LA, Geffner ME, Danoff TM, Gould E, Thornton PS. Random unstimulated pediatric luteinizing hormone levels are not reliable in the assessment of pubertal suppression during histrelin implant therapy. *Int J Pediatr Endocrinol.* 2013;2013(1):20. https://doi.org/10.1186/1687-9856-2013-20.

31. Boot AM, De Muinck Keizer-Schrama S, Pols HA, Krenning EP, Drop SL. Bone mineral density and body composition before and during treatment with gonadotropin-releasing hormone agonist in children with central precocious and early puberty. *J Clin Endocrinol Metab.* 1998;83(2):370−373. https://doi.org/10.1210/jcem.83.2.4573.

32. Lewis KA, Eugster EA. Random luteinizing hormone often remains pubertal in children treated with the histrelin implant for central precocious puberty. *J Pediatr.* 2013;162(3):562−565. https://doi.org/10.1016/j.jpeds.2012.08.038.

33. Neely EK, Wilson DM, Lee PA, Stene M, Hintz RL. Spontaneous serum gonadotropin concentrations in the evaluation of precocious puberty. *J Pediatr.* 1995; 127(1):47−52. http://www.ncbi.nlm.nih.gov/pubmed/7608810.

34. Neely EK, Lee PA, Bloch CA, et al. Leuprolide acetate 1-month depot for central precocious puberty: hormonal suppression and recovery. *Int J Pediatr Endocrinol.* 2010; 2010:1−9. https://doi.org/10.1155/2010/398639.

35. Silverman LA, Neely EK, Kletter GB, et al. Long-term continuous suppression with once-yearly histrelin subcutaneous implants for the treatment of central precocious puberty: a final report of a phase 3 multicenter trial. *J Clin Endocrinol Metab.* 2015;100(6):2354−2363. https://doi.org/10.1210/jc.2014-3031.

36. Zung A, Burundukov E, Ulman M, Glaser T, Zadik Z. Monitoring gonadotropin-releasing hormone analogue (GnRHa) treatment in girls with central precocious puberty: a comparison of four methods. *J Pediatr Endocrinol Metab.* 2015;28(7−8):885−893. https://doi.org/10.1515/jpem-2014-0478.

37. Brito VN, Batista MC, Borges MF, et al. Diagnostic value of fluorometric assays in the evaluation of precocious puberty. *J Clin Endocrinol Metab.* 1999;84(10): 3539−3544. https://doi.org/10.1210/jcem.84.10.6024.

38. Ibáñez L, Potau N, Zampolli M, et al. Use of leuprolide acetate response patterns in the early diagnosis of pubertal disorders: comparison with the gonadotropin-releasing hormone test. *J Clin Endocrinol Metab.* 1994;78(1): 30−35. https://doi.org/10.1210/jcem.78.1.7507123.

39. Eugster EA, Clarke W, Kletter GB, et al. Efficacy and safety of histrelin subdermal implant in children with central precocious puberty: a multicenter trial. *J Clin Endocrinol Metab.* 2007;92(5):1697−1704. https://doi.org/10.1210/jc.2006-2479.

40. Bhatia S, Neely EK, Wilson DM. Serum luteinizing hormone rises within minutes after depot leuprolide injection: implications for monitoring therapy. *Pediatrics.* 2002;109(2):E30. http://www.ncbi.nlm.nih.gov/pubmed/11826240.

41. Mouat F, Hofman PL, Jefferies C, Gunn AJ, Cutfield WS. Initial growth deceleration during GnRH analogue therapy for precocious puberty. *Clin Endocrinol (Oxf).* 2009;70(5):751−756. https://doi.org/10.1111/j.1365-2265.2008.03433.x.

42. Misra M, Pacaud D, Petryk A, Collett-Solberg PF, Kappy M, Drug and Therapeutics Committee of the Lawson Wilkins Pediatric Endocrine Society. Vitamin D deficiency in children and its management: review of current knowledge and recommendations. *Pediatrics.* 2008;122(2):398−417. https://doi.org/10.1542/peds.2007-1894.

43. Crabtree NJ, Arabi A, Bachrach LK, et al. Dual-energy x-ray absorptiometry interpretation and reporting in children and adolescents: the revised 2013 ISCD pediatric official positions. *J Clin Densitom.* 2014;17(2):225−242. https://doi.org/10.1016/j.jocd.2014.01.003.

CHAPTER 6

Psychosocial Considerations in Pubertal Suppression Treatment

DIANE CHEN, PHD • JENNIFER M. BIRNKRANT, MA • MARCO A. HIDALGO, PHD

INTRODUCTION

The last decade has marked a significant shift in the practice of pediatric transgender healthcare from regarding diverse gender identities and behaviors as inherently pathological and necessitating corrective "treatment" toward affirming youth's gender identities, expressions, and related experiences. Clinical practice guidelines have been established based on the collective expertise of clinicians working with transgender and gender-nonconforming (TGNC) youth and are rapidly evolving, in many cases outpacing outcomes research. Medical treatments like pubertal suppression (e.g., "puberty blockers") with gonadotropin-releasing hormone analogues (GnRHa) have been used with TGNC youth for over 20 years[1] and is now considered the standard of care for peripubertal TGNC youth with gender dysphoria (i.e., the affective distress that arises from incongruence between one's gender identity and assigned sex at birth).[2–4] GnRHa is considered a fully reversible treatment that allows for a temporary suspension in the development of secondary sex characteristics. This "pausing" of pubertal development affords youth in the early stages of puberty the opportunity for an extended period of ongoing gender exploration, without the affective distress associated with unwanted pubertal development. For youth who later decide to initiate gender-affirming estrogen or testosterone, GnRHa treatment facilitates a physical transition that minimizes the need for more invasive, surgical interventions. For youth who decide not to pursue physical gender transition, discontinuing GnRHa will allow reactivation of the hypothalamic–pituitary–gonadal axis, leading to a resumption of one's endogenous puberty.[5]

The few studies examining the psychosocial outcomes of pubertal suppression have demonstrated that youth receiving pubertal suppression treatment show significant reductions in depression symptoms and improvement in overall psychosocial functioning.[6,7] In one study, the proportion of youth scoring in the clinical range on reliable parent report measures of internalizing and externalizing behaviors decreased from 44% to 22% from baseline (prior to GnRHa treatment) to initiation of gender-affirming hormones (an average of 2 years following GnRHa initiation).[7] Given these positive psychosocial outcomes and the presumed reversibility of treatment, GnRHa is often presented as a benign treatment that "buys time" for TGNC youth to either further explore gender identity or to further mature before having to make a decision about medical interventions that are partially irreversible in nature. However, there has been some debate regarding whether GnRHa is truly reversible, with some arguing that certain psychosocial risks or "side effects" warrant consideration in decision-making about pubertal suppression treatment. The goal of this chapter is to highlight these psychosocial considerations in pubertal suppression treatment. To this end, we review the following: (1) controversy surrounding the possible effects of pubertal suppression treatment on gender identity and/or sexuality development, (2) unknown neurocognitive sequelae of pubertal suppression treatment, (3) psychosocial implications of medical side effects, including GnRHa effects on future fertility and sexual functioning, and (4) family factors related to GnRHa treatment.

POSSIBLE EFFECTS OF GONADOTROPIN-RELEASING HORMONE ANALOGUES ON GENDER IDENTITY AND/OR SEXUALITY DEVELOPMENT

There has been recent debate around whether suppressing a child's endogenous puberty may result in iatrogenic effects that alter the "natural course" of that child's gender identity development and formation.[8,9]

For example, Giordano has argued that experiencing one's own endogenous puberty may serve an important function in clarifying questions or concerns about one's own body and gender identity.[9] This argument, referred to as a "crisis of gender," suggests that it is necessary for TGNC youth to be initially exposed to the development of natal secondary sex characteristics before making the crucial determination regarding whether or not pubertal development is aversive and distressing.[9] The concern is that suppressing endogenous puberty using GnRHa may prevent youth from critically evaluating the degree of distress associated with the physical changes of their endogenous puberty and result in the persistence of gender dysphoria which may not have otherwise persisted.[10]

Similarly, Stein expressed concern that pubertal suppression treatment in early adolescence may be the strongest predictor in the eventual uptake of gender-affirming hormones and surgical intervention.[11] He posits that the use of GnRHa, while often considered a way to "buy time" before making decisions about partially irreversible treatments, may actually push adolescents down a path toward additional medical interventions. Stein notes that because we do not know how pubertal suppression treatment affects TGNC youths' gender identity development, its use "may not necessarily maximize life options—it may close off some options by keeping others open."[11] However, he acknowledges that these concerns are speculative and that the risks of nonintervention must be weighed against the unknowns of intervention.

While acknowledging similar concerns, Cohen-Kettenis and colleagues have reported on their clinical observation of youth from the Netherlands that gender dysphoria persisting after pubertal onset is unlikely to remit.[12] Adolescents deemed eligible for medical intervention at the Netherlands clinic have continued to affirm a transgender identity and have not expressed regret related to gender-affirming treatment. In addition, it was not until 2007 that the first multidisciplinary pediatric gender clinic was formally established in the United States,[13] and the option for medical transition for youth has been more widely accessible. Thus, transgender individuals have historically pursued medical transition in adulthood, after progressing fully through their endogenous puberty, which demonstrates that exposure to one's endogenous hormones does not necessarily result in the development of a cisgender identity.

Similar to concerns about altered gender identity development and consolidation, others have raised the possibility that pubertal suppression treatment

may impact the course of a child's psychosexual development.[8,14] It has been suggested that suppressing endogenous puberty may delay normative, age-appropriate sexual exploration and sexual identity development as a result of not being exposed to increasing levels of sex hormones (i.e., testosterone or estrogen) that are typical during puberty.[8] While there is some agreement that the implications of pubertal suppression on sexuality require more study and attention,[7] no published research has examined this theoretical concern to date.

Korte et al. have also proposed the possibility that pubertal suppression treatment may mask internalized homophobia and rejection of same-sex attraction in some youth.[8] In their Berlin-based gender clinic, the authors observed a handful of youth initially referred for gender dysphoria whose dysphoria ultimately resolved as they identified a primarily same-sex attraction. Korte et al. assert that these youth may have experienced an initial desire to transition due to internalized homophobia and wanting to identify as heterosexual.[8] Therefore, pubertal suppression treatment in these patients may inadvertently serve to increase identity confusion, reinforce internalized homophobia, and interfere with youths' natural sexual identity formation.[8]

Still others have raised concern that pubertal suppression treatment may not only hinder the natural course of gender identity and/or sexuality development but also result in a global stunting of typical adolescent personal growth. Giovanardi contends that pubertal suppression treatment may "disconnect" an adolescent from typical experiences that are critical to identity formation; he suggests that pubertal suppression may result in youth not experiencing an adolescence, which is typically regarded as a time of self-exploration and experimentation.[14] He summarizes that "the main dilemma is to understand whether buying time at such a precocious age truly enables children to explore deep personal meanings, or whether it freezes youngsters in a prolonged childhood, secluding them from certain aspects of reality and isolating them from peer groups."[14] However, it should be noted there is no empirical evidence to support this theoretical concern.

It is also possible that youth who undergo pubertal suppression treatment may experience distress or continued dysphoria due to having a body that appears prepubescent (while peers may develop typically). In a prospective follow-up study of 70 youth undergoing pubertal suppression treatment in the Netherlands, youth did not experience significant remittance of gender dysphoria or dissatisfaction with primary and secondary sex characteristics after an average of 2 years of pubertal suppression treatment.[7] Although these results do not indicate adverse outcomes of pubertal suppression per se, it should be noted that pubertal suppression may not result in significant reductions in gender-related distress, likely because GnRHa does not result in phenotypical changes consistent with a youth's affirmed gender.[15] However, although gender dysphoria and body dissatisfaction did not improve, youth experienced significant reductions in depressive symptoms and significant improvements in overall psychosocial functioning over the course of treatment, which suggests pubertal suppression treatment alone may have overall positive effects on youths' global psychological and behavioral functioning.[7]

UNKNOWN NEUROCOGNITIVE SEQUELAE OF PUBERTAL SUPPRESSION TREATMENT

A commonly cited unknown side effect of pubertal suppression treatment pertains to the impact of GnRHa on neurocognitive development. It is well documented that adolescence represents a developmental period associated with profound changes in physical and social maturation, and also with significant gains in neurocognitive development.[16,17] Structural and functional aspects of brain development during early adolescence point to significant growth and change in the prefrontal cortex, especially with respect to myelination and synaptic pruning processes that result in increased efficiency of information processing.[18,19] These changes are thought to underlie various aspects of executive functioning, including long-term planning, meta cognition, self-evaluation, self-regulation, and the coordination of affect and cognition.[20]

In addition, adolescence also represents a time of improved connectivity between regions of the prefrontal cortex and several areas of the limbic system. Steinberg argues that this restructuring creates a context in which changes in an adolescent's arousal and motivation precede the development of regulatory competence, creating "a disjunction between the adolescent's affective experience and his or her ability to regulate arousal and motivation."[17] These widespread structural and functional changes in adolescent brain development that occur during puberty begs the question of the extent to which sex hormones (i.e., estrogen and testosterone which are considered "pubertal hormones") play a role in neurocognitive development during this critical period.

Relatively little is known about the relationship between the biological process of puberty (i.e., exposure to sex hormones) and neurocognitive development in humans. However, research in nonhuman animal studies have found that hormonal exposure during puberty exerts profound effects on brain maturation and behavior.[21,22] In these studies, sex hormones exert three main effects on behavior at puberty via distinct brain regions (see Blakemore et al., 2010 for review).[23] First, sex hormones impact reproductive behaviors, which mainly occur via the hypothalamus.[23] Second, sex hormones impact the reorganization of sensory and association regions of the brain, resulting in altered sensory associations that may facilitate attentional and motivational changes at puberty. Last, sex hormones affect the nucleus accumbens and the dopaminergic pathways to the prefrontal cortex, resulting in effects to the reward centers of the brain.[23]

The advent of noninvasive brain imaging techniques has enabled the study of human brain development during puberty. Human neuroimaging studies have consistently found that in typically developing pubertal children, cortical and subcortical gray matter decreases, whereas white matter increases throughout puberty.[23] There is also some evidence that sex hormones may play a direct role in adolescent brain development.[23] This introduces the possibility that suppressing sex hormone production during the early stages of puberty may result in negative neurocognitive sequelae.

To date, two studies have directly explored the impact of pubertal suppression treatment on neurocognitive development among peripubertal transgender youth. First, Staphorsius and colleagues examined whether performance on the Tower of London task (ToL), a commonly used neuropsychological test of executive functioning, was altered in transgender youth when treated with GnRHa.[24] Researchers found no significant effect of GnRHa on ToL performance scores—i.e., reaction times and accuracy—when comparing GnRHa-treated transgender girls with untreated transgender girls or when comparing GnRHa-treated transgender boys with untreated transgender boys.[24] A second case study examined the effects of pubertal suppression treatment on brain white matter and cognitive functioning. Schneider and colleagues conducted a longitudinal evaluation of a pubertal transgender girl undergoing GnRHa treatment for pubertal suppression with three longitudinal magnetic resonance imaging scans and cognitive assessments using the Wechsler Intelligence Scale (WISC-IV).[25] She was evaluated at baseline, before GnRHa initiation, and at 22 and 28 months post-GnRHa treatment. During the follow-up period, white matter fractional anisotropy did not increase, compared to expected normal male puberty effects on the brain. After 22 months of pubertal suppression treatment, working memory scores on the WISC-IV dropped 9 points and remained stable after 28 months of follow-up.[25] The authors concluded that normative increases in brain white matter appeared disrupted in this transgender girl on pubertal suppression treatment; she also exhibited a reduction in working memory scores on the WISC-IV, which affected her global cognitive functioning, while on pubertal suppression treatment.

There remain many questions regarding the functional and structural effects of pubertal suppression treatment on neurocognitive development in transgender youth treated with GnRHa, with conflicting findings in two studies measuring distinct aspects of neurocognitive development using differing research designs. Thus, the potential for pubertal suppression treatment to be associated with negative side effects impacting neurocognitive development should be discussed with youth and families during the consent process for GnRHa initiation. The unknown risk of GnRHa on neurocognitive development should be weighed against the known benefits of pubertal suppression treatment on overall psychosocial and behavioral functioning.[7]

PSYCHOSOCIAL IMPLICATIONS OF KNOWN MEDICAL SIDE EFFECTS OF GONADOTROPIN-RELEASING HORMONE ANALOGUE TREATMENT

Fertility Considerations

The World Professional Association of Transgender Health Standards of Care, Version 7[4] and the 2009 Endocrine Society Clinical Practice Guidelines[2] both recommend counseling regarding fertility and fertility preservation options for transgender individuals prior to initiating gender-affirming hormone treatment in recognition of research suggesting that long-term hormone treatment may lead to impairments in gonadal histology that cause infertility or biological sterility.[26–29] However, the evolving standards of transgender healthcare emphasizes the need to address fertility earlier in the care continuum, as pubertal suppression treatment with GnRHa not only prevents the development of unwanted secondary sex characteristics but also suspends germ cell maturation.[30] While GnRHa treatment represents a reversible intervention, in that puberty appears to progress normally after discontinuing GnRHa,[31] the vast majority of transgender youth initiate gender-affirming testosterone or estrogen concurrently with GnRHa or before discontinuing GnRHa.[3] Youth who initiate gender-affirming hormones concurrently with GnRHa, or prior to discontinuing GnRHa, will not

have the opportunity to pursue nonexperimental oocyte or sperm cryopreservation. While procedures exist to preserve prepubertal ovarian or testicular tissue, these fertility preservation techniques are considered experimental and must be conducted within the confines of an approved institutional review board protocol,[32] thus limiting access to care.

As pubertal suppression treatment has become the standard of care, the revised Endocrine Society Clinical Practice Guidelines[33] now recommends counseling regarding fertility prior to pubertal suppression initiation. This means that TGNC youth, who may be as young as 8–9 years in the early stages of puberty, may be put in a position to consider their future parenting desires and intentions during a developmental period when it is nonnormative to be considering family planning decisions. It is possible that introducing these topics to a young adolescent who does not possess the emotional maturity to consider their fertility and parenting intentions may result in distress or confusion.

Moreover, pediatric fertility preservation options and the assisted reproductive technologies necessary to utilize cryopreserved tissue are complex and rapidly evolving. Thus, it may be difficult for transgender healthcare providers to effectively and accurately counsel early pubertal youth and their parents on the available options and ensure families fully understand the fertility implications of pubertal suppression treatment without providing referrals to fertility specialists. However, a recent study demonstrates that transgender youth rarely seek additional fertility counseling outside of their primary, gender-affirming treatment team, despite routine discussion about the availability of specialized fertility counseling.[34] In the context of impending pubertal changes that are causing significant distress, it is not only possible, but likely that youth may prioritize short-term needs (e.g., suppressing puberty and distressing pubertal changes) over the potential for long-term consequences (e.g., decisional regret about compromised fertility). This is particularly problematic as impaired fertility affects future quality of life,[35–37] rather than current functioning or survival. Thus, the psychosocial impact of impaired fertility may be unknown until adulthood.

Sexual Function Considerations

As highlighted by Mahfouda and colleagues, the decision to suppression endogenous puberty has implications on later gender-affirming surgical interventions.[15] Specifically, vaginectomy in a transgender man requires surgical reconstruction of the vaginal mucosa and labia—procedures which are associated with a high risk of postoperative bleeding and urological complications.[38] Estrogen plays an important role in the structural integrity of vaginal tissue and proliferation of the epithelium, posing challenges for transmen who have had little exposure to estrogen due to pubertal suppression treatment in early adolescence.[15] In addition, the most common surgical technique for creating a neovagina for transgender women—a penile inversion vaginoplasty—requires sufficient phallic and scrotal development, corresponding with Tanner stage 4 genital development.[39,40] Transwomen treated with GnRHa in early puberty may, therefore, be limited in their options for later gender-affirming genital surgery. While other surgical options exist, such as laparoscopic intestinal vaginoplasty with the sigmoid colon, clinically observed risks include postcoital bleeding, and potentially compromising sexual functioning in adulthood.[39] Similar to fertility-related psychosocial considerations, any impairment to sexual functioning as a direct result of GnRHa treatment will remain unknown until youth reach late adolescence or adulthood. At the point in development during which peripubertal transgender youth are making decisions about GnRHa treatment, they are unlikely to understand the implications of decreased sexual functioning on future quality of life.

FAMILY FACTORS

There is a growing body of evidence documenting the positive impact of supportive parenting on TGNC youth development. For instance, Olson and colleagues found that socially transitioned prepubertal children—those who were supported in living in their affirmed gender roles by their families—exhibited normative levels of depressive symptoms and minimally increased anxiety symptoms, and overall much lower internalizing symptomology than previous reports in nontransitioned youth with gender dysphoria.[41,42] Increased gender affirmation and parental support for transition is also associated with decreased depression and suicide attempts in transgender teens and young adults.[43]

While affirming parents can serve as a protective factor and positively impact psychosocial functioning among TGNC youth, parents also control access to medical treatment, particularly for early pubertal youth who are eligible for pubertal suppression treatment. In a study of transgender youths' perspectives on barriers to gender-affirming healthcare, participants frequently identified lack of family approval as a barrier to treatment, particularly among those youth that relied on a caregivers' insurance plan to pay for treatment.[44] The lack of support for GnRHa by parents as well as the lack of consensus *between* parents regarding GnRHa

treatment may lead to significant conflict and stress for TGNC youth. Tishelman and colleagues note that it is particularly challenging when two parents or guardians with shared medical decision-making rights are in disagreement about how or whether to proceed with medical transition.[45] Given that parental consensus is often needed to proceed with pubertal suppression treatment, multidisciplinary gender health teams may need to support families in navigating difficult discussions and decisions.

Finally, pubertal suppression treatment is variably covered by insurance plans and may lead to significant financial burden for families with out-of-pocket costs ranging from $120 to $1000 per month.[45] Nahata and colleagues report that insurance coverage for gender-affirming medical interventions may range from less than 20% to approximately 70% across medical centers serving transgender youth in the United States.[46] Insurance exclusions were identified as a barrier to accessing gender-affirming treatments, with some families ultimately withdrawing their child from care after discovering that their insurance plans did not cover gender-affirming care.[44] Ehrensaft explains frankly that the price tag associated with GnRHa treatment, if not covered by medical insurance or government programs, is out of reach for all except those with substantial financial means.[47] Facing these significant and real financial barriers to care may contribute to TGNC youth viewing their parents as unsupportive or even rejecting, potentially causing additional stress for the child and for the family as a whole.[48]

CONCLUSION

Pubertal suppression treatment is widely recognized as the standard of care for peripubertal TGNC youth with gender dysphoria. Historically considered a "fully reversible" treatment with documented benefits on psychosocial functioning, the potential psychosocial risks or "side effects" associated with GnRHa are less often discussed compared to risks associated with gender-affirming estrogen or testosterone. In this chapter, we have highlighted the key psychosocial considerations in pubertal suppression treatment. Important to note, many of these considerations focus on theoretical risks (e.g., possible effects of pubertal suppression treatment on gender identity development and consolidation) or unknown risks (e.g., unknown neurocognitive sequelae of pubertal suppression treatment), which must be considered in the context of the known psychosocial benefits of GnRHa treatment on TGNC youth with gender dysphoria when making decisions about appropriate gender-affirming medical care.

REFERENCES

1. Cohen-Kettenis PT, van Goozen SH. Pubertal delay as an aid in diagnosis and treatment of a transsexual adolescent. *Eur Child Adolesc Psychiatry.* 1998;7(4):246−248.
2. Hembree WC, Cohen-Kettenis P, Delemarre-van de Waal HA, et al. Endocrine treatment of transsexual persons: an Endocrine Society clinical practice guideline. *J Clin Endocrinol Metab.* 2009;94(9):3132−3154.
3. Hembree WC. Guidelines for pubertal suspension and gender reassignment for transgender adolescents. *Child Adolesc Psychiatr Clin N Am.* 2011;20(4):725−732.
4. Coleman E, Bockting W, Botzer M, et al. Standards of care for the health of transsexual,transgender, and gender-nonconforming people, Version 7. *Int J Transgenderism.* 2012;13:165−232.
5. de Vries AL, Cohen-Kettenis PT. Clinical management of gender dysphoria in children and adolescents: the Dutch approach. *J Homosex.* 2012;59(3):301−320.
6. Costa R, Dunsford M, Skagerberg E, Holt V, Carmichael P, Colizzi M. Psychological support, puberty suppression, and psychosocial functioning in adolescents with gender dysphoria. *J Sex Med.* 2015;12(11):2206−2214.
7. de Vries AL, Steensma TD, Doreleijers TA, Cohen-Kettenis PT. Puberty suppression in adolescents with gender identity disorder: a prospective follow-up study. *J Sex Med.* 2011;8(8):2276−2283.
8. Korte A, Lehmkuhl U, Goecker D, Beier KM, Krude H, Gruters-Kieslich A. Gender identity disorders in childhood and adolescence: currently debated concepts and treatment strategies. *Dtsch Arztebl Int.* 2008;105(48):834−841.
9. Giordano S. Gender atypical organisation in children and adolescents: ethico-legal Issues and a proposal for new guidelines. *Int J Chil Rights.* 2007;15(3):365−390.
10. Vrouenraets LJJJ, Fredriks AM, Hannema SE, Cohen-Kettenis PT, de Vries MC. Early medical treatment of children and adolescents with gender dysphoria: an empirical ethical study. *J Adolesc Health.* 2015;57(4):367−373.
11. Stein E. Commentary on the treatment of gender variant and gender dysphoric children and adolescents: common themes and ethical reflections. *J Homosex.* 2012;59(3):480−500.
12. Cohen-Kettenis PT, Steensma TD, de Vries ALC. Treatment of adolescents with gender dysphoria in The Netherlands. *Child Adolesc Psychiatr Clin N Am.* 2011;20(4):689−700.
13. Edwards-Leeper L, Spack NP. Psychological evaluation and medical treatment of transgender youth in an interdisciplinary "Gender Management Service" (GeMS) in a major pediatric center. *J Homosex.* 2012;59(3):321−336.
14. Giovanardi G. Buying time or arresting development? The dilemma of administering hormone blockers in trans children and adolescents. *Porto Biomed J.* 2017;2(5):153−156.
15. Mahfouda S, Moore JK, Siafarikas A, Zepf FD, Lin A. Puberty suppression in transgender children and adolescents. *Lancet Diabetes Endocrinol.* 2017;5(10):816−826.
16. Paus T. Mapping brain maturation and cognitive development during adolescence. *Trends Cogn Sci.* 2005;9(2):60−68.
17. Steinberg L. Cognitive and affective development in adolescence. *Trends Cogn Sci.* 2005;9(2):69−74.
18. Sowell ER, Trauner DA, Gamst A, Jernigan TL. Development of cortical and subcortical brain structures in childhood and adolescence: a structural MRI study. *Dev Med Child Neurol.* 2002;44(1):4−16.
19. Paus T, Zijdenbos A, Worsley K, et al. Structural maturation of neural pathways in children and adolescents: in vivo study. *Science.* 1999;283(5409):1908−1911.
20. Keating DP. Cognitive and brain development. In: Lerner RM, Steinberg L, Lerner RM, Steinberg L, eds. *Handbook of Adolescent Psychology.* Hoboken, NJ: John Wiley & Sons Inc; 2004:45−84.
21. Spear LP. The adolescent brain and age-related behavioral manifestations. *Neurosci Biobehav Rev.* 2000;24(4):417−463.
22. Sisk CL, Foster DL. The neural basis of puberty and adolescence. *Nat Neurosci.* 2004;7(10):1040−1047.
23. Blakemore SJ, Burnett S, Dahl RE. The role of puberty in the developing adolescent brain. *Hum Brain Mapp.* 2010;31(6):926−933.
24. Staphorsius AS, Kreukels BP, Cohen-Kettenis PT, et al. Puberty suppression and executive functioning: an fMRI-study in adolescents with gender dysphoria. *Psychoneuroendocrinology.* 2015;56:190−199.
25. Schneider MA, Spritzer PM, Soll BMB, et al. Brain maturation, cognition and voice pattern in a gender dysphoria case under pubertal suppression. *Front Hum Neurosci.* 2017;11:528.
26. Ikeda K, Baba T, Noguchi H, et al. Excessive androgen exposure in female-to-male transsexual persons of reproductive age induces hyperplasia of the ovarian cortex and stroma but not polycystic ovary morphology. *Hum Reprod.* 2013;28(2):453−461.
27. Lubbert H, Leo-Rossberg I, Hammerstein J. Effects of ethinyl estradiol on semen quality and various hormonal parameters in a eugonadal male. *Fertil Steril.* 1992;58(3):603−608.
28. Pache TD, Chadha S, Gooren LJ, et al. Ovarian morphology in long-term androgen-treated female to male transsexuals. A human model for the study of polycystic ovarian syndrome? *Histopathology.* 1991;19(5):445−452.
29. Schulze C. Response of the human testis to long-term estrogen treatment: morphology of Sertoli cells, Leydig cells and spermatogonial stem cells. *Cell Tissue Res.* 1988;251(1):31−43.
30. Johnson EK, Finlayson C. Preservation of fertility potential for gender and sex diverse individuals. *Transgend Health.* 2016;1(1):41−44.
31. Hagen CP, Sorensen K, Anderson RA, Juul A. Serum levels of antimullerian hormone in early maturing girls before, during, and after suppression with GnRH agonist. *Fertil Steril.* 2012;98(5):1326−1330.
32. Johnson EK, Finlayson C, Rowell EE, et al. Fertility preservation for pediatric patients: current state and future possibilities. *J Urol.* 2017;198(1):186−194.

33. Hembree WC, Cohen-Kettenis PT, Gooren L, et al. Endocrine treatment of gender-dysphoric/gender-incongruent persons: an endocrine society clinical practice guideline. *J Clin Endocrinol Metab*. 2017.

34. Chen D, Simons L, Johnson EK, Lockart BA, Finlayson C. Fertility preservation for transgender adolescents. *J Adolesc Health*. 2017;61(1):120−123.

35. Smith NK, Madeira J, Millard HR. Sexual function and fertility quality of life in women using in vitro fertilization. *J Sex Med*. 2015;12(4):985−993.

36. Canada AL, Schover LR. The psychosocial impact of interrupted childbearing in long-term female cancer survivors. *Psychooncology*. 2012;21(2):134−143.

37. Nilsson J, Jervaeus A, Lampic C, et al. 'Will I be able to have a baby?' Results from online focus group discussions with childhood cancer survivors in Sweden. *Hum Reprod*. 2014; 29(12):2704−2711.

38. Cagnacci A, Piacenti I, Zanin R, Xholli A, Tirelli A. Influence of an oral contraceptive containing drospirenone on insulin sensitivity of healthy women. *Eur J Obstet Gynecol Reprod Biol*. 2014;178:48−50.

39. Schechter LS. Gender confirmation surgery: an update for the primary care provider. *Transgend Health*. 2016;1(1):32−40.

40. Colebunders B, Brondeel S, D'Arpa S, Hoebeke P, Monstrey S. An update on the surgical treatment for transgender patients. *Sex Med Rev*. 2017;5(1):103−109.

41. Olson KR, Durwood L, DeMeules M, McLaughlin KA. Mental health of transgender children who are supported in their identities. *Pediatrics*. 2016;137(3):e20153223.

42. Durwood L, McLaughlin KA, Olson KR. Mental health and self-worth in socially transitioned transgender youth. *J Am Acad Child Adolesc Psychiatry*. 2017;56(2):116−123.e112.

43. Travers R, Bauer G, Pyne J, Bradley K, Gale L, Papadimitriou M. *Impacts of Strong Parental Support for Trans Youth: A Report Prepared for Children's Aid Society of Toronto and Delisle Youth Services*. 2012.

44. Gridley SJ, Crouch JM, Evans Y, et al. Youth and caregiver perspectives on barriers to gender-affirming health care for transgender youth. *J Adolesc Health*. 2016;59(3):254−261.

45. Tishelman AC, Kaufman R, Edwards-Leeper L, Mandel FH, Shumer DE, Spack NP. Serving transgender youth: challenges, dilemmas and clinical examples. *Prof Psychol Res Pr*. 2015;46(1):37−45.

46. Nahata L, Chelvakumar G, Leibowitz S. Gender-affirming pharmacological interventions for youth with gender dysphoria: when treatment guidelines are not enough. *Ann Pharmacother*. 2017;51(11):1023−1032.

47. Ehrensaft D. Look, Mom, I'm a boy—don't tell anyone I was a girl. *J LGBT Youth*. 2013;10(1−2):9−28.

48. Leibowitz SF, Spack NP. The development of a gender identity psychosocial clinic: treatment issues, logistical considerations, interdisciplinary cooperation, and future initiatives. *Child Adolesc Psychiatr Clin N Am*. 2011;20(4): 701−724.

CHAPTER 7

Medical Side Effects of GnRH Agonists

LIAT PERL, MD[a] • JANET Y. LEE, MD, MPH[a] • STEPHEN M. ROSENTHAL, MD

Based on pioneering work from the Netherlands, the Endocrine Society (ES) Clinical Practice Guidelines and World Professional Association for Transgender Health (WPATH) Standards of Care endorse the use of pubertal blockers using gonadotropin-releasing hormone (GnRH) agonists not before Tanner stage 2 in individuals experiencing either the emergence or a significant increase in gender dysphoria with the onset of puberty.[1,2] While currently available mental health outcomes data support these ES and WPATH recommendations,[3] there are potential adverse effects of pubertal suppression in gender dysphoric youth treated with GnRH agonists, including impaired bone mineralization, compromised fertility, and unclear effects on brain development, body mass index (BMI), and body composition.

BONE HEALTH

Given that peak bone mass is achieved during puberty and young adulthood, pubertal suppression with GnRH agonists at Tanner 2 or later could impair bone mineralization, particularly if there is a prolonged period of hypogonadism.[4] While the initial ES Clinical Practice Guidelines recommended waiting until the age of 16 years to initiate sex hormone treatment in pubertally suppressed transgender youth,[5] the recently revised guidelines recognize that there may be compelling reasons (e.g., preservation of bone health) to initiate cross-sex hormone treatment before the age of 16 years, and thereby limit the period of hypogonadism.[1] The skeletal consequences of pubertal suppression in early pubertal gender dysphoric youth have yet to be rigorously studied, but existing literature, based on protocols summarized in the initial ES guidelines, raise substantial concerns.

Peak bone mass, achieved during puberty and young adulthood, is a major determinant of future adult fracture risk.[4,6] Late menarche is associated with impaired bone microstructure and increased fracture risk during childhood and adolescence, during which there already is a baseline increased incidence of fracture.[4] There is evidence that the age of onset of puberty does predict bone mass in young adulthood, but adequate long-term follow-up data are lacking.[7] Some studies of adult men indicate lower bone mineral density (BMD) in those with delayed puberty when compared with men with normal timing of puberty,[8–11] while others have shown no difference.[12,13] Whether these differences in BMD result in change in fracture risk has not been definitively investigated in men.[14] Individuals with central precocious puberty treated with GnRH agonists experience a dip in BMD at the onset of pubertal suppression, but levels rebound to control values after discontinuation of GnRH agonists, when endogenous puberty resumes.[15]

Few studies have examined bone health in transgender youth, but data from European groups have indicated that transgender women have a propensity toward lower BMD at baseline prior to any cross-hormone therapy.[16,17] In transgender youth, bone data from the Netherlands were reported in adolescents who had reached a later stage of puberty (Tanner 4–5) at the time of initiation of pubertal suppression, with a mean age of 14.9–15 years, followed by initiation of cross-sex hormone therapy around 16 years of age, and who several years later ultimately underwent gonadectomy.[18] This cohort showed lower baseline BMD z-scores in the transgender girls prior to any gender-affirming medical treatment. Median duration of GnRH agonist monotherapy was 1.3 years in transgender females and 1.5 years in transgender males. As expected, BMD z-scores in both the transgender females and males fell during GnRH agonist monotherapy, but the transgender adolescent females did not recover their BMD z-scores after a median duration of 5.8 years of gender-affirming estrogen therapy.[18]

Another study from the Netherlands investigated bone turnover markers and BMD in transgender adolescents stratified by younger (bone age <15 years in

---

[a]Contributed equally

transgender girls or <14 years in transgender boys) or older (bone age ≥15 years in transgender girls or ≥14 years in transgender boys) age groups.[19] These transgender adolescents underwent treatment with GnRH agonists followed by gender-affirming hormone therapy at the age of 16 years similar to previous reports.[18] At baseline, bone mineral apparent density (BMAD) in the lumbar spine was lower in young transgender female adolescents versus young transgender male adolescents. Following GnRH agonist treatment, bone turnover markers and BMAD z-scores decreased in the younger groups, and 24 months of cross-sex hormone treatment led to an increase in BMAD in all groups.[19]

It has been postulated that transgender girls may be less active than their cisgender boy peers. Although weight-bearing exercise is a significant factor in BMD,[6] as are dietary calcium and vitamin D levels, these data were not reported in the published studies. Additionally, both studies of transgender adolescents showed an expected drop in BMD z-scores during pubertal suppression that, in the confines of the particular studies, did not recover to baseline after estradiol therapy in most transgender girls.[18,19]

A 22-year follow-up of the first described gender dysphoric adolescent treated with GnRH agonist and subsequent cross-sex hormones reported that BMD was within the normal range for both sexes.[20] This individual was treated with GnRH agonist from 13.7 years until 18.6 years of age before initiating cross-sex hormone treatment, with BMD z-scores reported at the age of 35 years.[20]

BRAIN

Puberty has been suggested to represent a second organizational period during brain development when remarkable remodeling of cortical and limbic circuits occurs. This critical period of neuronal development and programming is thought to lead to the acquisition of adult cognition, decision-making strategies, and social behaviors. Some of this organizational processing is thought to be linked to the elevation of gonadal hormones, which occurs during puberty.[21]

Furthermore, GnRH receptor expression and GnRH binding are present in extrapituitary tissues, including brain regions such as the hippocampus and other limbic structures, indicating that GnRH might have a direct effect on brain function outside the hypothalamic–pituitary–gonadal (HPG) axis.[22] Long-term GnRH agonist treatment in transgender adolescents initiated in early puberty, therefore, raises concerns regarding potential cognitive and behavioral effects, due to the blockade of GnRH signaling within and outside the HPG axis.

A recent study in an ovine model assessed spatial maze performance and memory in rams that were untreated (controls), had both GnRH and testosterone signaling blocked (GnRH agonist-treated), or specifically had GnRH signaling blocked (GnRH agonist-treated with testosterone replacement) during the peripubertal period.[22] The results demonstrated that emotional reactivity (emotional and behavioral responses to a fearful situation) during spatial tasks was compromised by the blockade of gonadal steroid signaling, as seen by the restorative effects of testosterone replacement.[22] The blockade of GnRH signaling alone was associated with impaired retention of long-term spatial memory, and this effect was not restored with the replacement of testosterone signaling.[22] Furthermore, a follow-up study demonstrated that the long-term spatial memory performance of rams that were treated with GnRH agonists in the peripubertal stage remained reduced after discontinuation of GnRH agonists.[23]

In humans, a study which assessed 15 cisgender girls with idiopathic central precocious puberty treated with GnRH agonists and 15 matched controls demonstrated that the treated girls displayed significantly higher emotional reactivity on one of two emotional reactivity task conditions.[24] Another study demonstrated a significant deterioration in performance on 2 tests of working memory function following 4 weeks of GnRH agonist treatment in 25 cisgender premenopausal women.[25]

In the transgender population, Schneider et al. performed a longitudinal evaluation of a pubertal transgender girl undergoing treatment with GnRH agonist.[26] They reported lack of significant variation in brain white matter fractional anisotropy, thought to be a measure of brain maturation, during pubertal suppression with GnRH agonist treatment for 28 months. They also reported a 9-point drop in operational memory tests after 22 months of pubertal suppression.[26] On the other hand, a cross-sectional study assessed executive functioning (performance on the Tower of London task) in adolescents with gender dysphoria when treated with GnRH agonists. The study showed no significant effect of GnRH agonists on performance scores between treated and untreated gender dysphoric adolescents.[27]

Further longitudinal clinical studies among transgender adolescents undergoing pubertal suppression are needed to assess the impact of GnRH agonist treatment on brain function and development.

FERTILITY

Transgender individuals often wish to preserve potential for fertility. It has been demonstrated in several studies that treatment with GnRH agonists in youth with central precocious puberty does not impair future fertility[15] and that frequency of pregnancy complications was comparable to controls.[28] Bertelloni et al. confirmed normal testicular function in adolescent boys after GnRH agonist therapy with full pubertal development and testicular volume, gonadotropins, testosterone, and inhibin B levels in the normal adult range.[12]

In the transgender population, however, if the use of GnRH agonists in early pubertal gender dysphoric children is later followed by treatment with cross-sex hormones, fertility will be compromised due to arrested gonadal maturation. Currently, experimental harvesting of prepubertal gonadal tissue, cryopreservation, and in vitro maturation are being explored in other medical contexts,[29,30] and may be of benefit for fertility preservation in early pubertal transgender youth. Research to obtain artificial gametes through stem cells is also ongoing and could be a feasible option in the future for those individuals who cannot or have not stored their own gametes.[31]

BODY MASS INDEX AND BODY COMPOSITION

Concern has been raised regarding the effect of GnRH agonist treatment on BMI and body composition in the transgender population, as previous studies in girls with precocious puberty demonstrated a slight increase in BMI during such treatment.[32] Other studies have shown no effect of GnRH agonist treatment on body composition or BMI.[33] In a study of 15 transgender female and 19 transgender male adolescents, treatment with GnRH agonist did not induce a change in BMI standard deviation score.[18] On the other hand, following GnRH agonist treatment, Schagen et al. observed an increase in fat percentage and decrease in lean body mass percentage in gender dysphoric adolescents (both transgender males and transgender females).[34]

SUMMARY

Further prospective studies focused on long-term safety and efficacy are necessary to optimize GnRH agonist treatment of transgender youth. Such studies pertain to the use of GnRH agonist both as a monotherapy in early pubertal gender dysphoric youth as well as longer-term use of GnRH agonist in combination with cross-sex hormones (in particular, in transgender females treated with estrogen) who have not undergone gonadectomy at the age of 18 years or later.

REFERENCES

1. Hembree WC, Cohen-Kettenis PT, Gooren L, et al. Endocrine treatment of gender-dysphoric/gender-incongruent persons: an endocrine society clinical practice guideline. *J Clin Endocrinol Metab.* 2017;102(11):3869−3903.
2. Coleman E, Bockting W, Botzer M, et al. Standards of care for the health of transsexual, transgender, and gender-nonconforming people, Version 7. *Int J Transgend.* 2012; 13(4):165−232.
3. de Vries AL, McGuire JK, Steensma TD, Wagenaar EC, Doreleijers TA, Cohen-Kettenis PT. Young adult psychological outcome after puberty suppression and gender reassignment. *Pediatrics.* 2014;134(4):696−704.
4. Bonjour JP, Chevalley T. Pubertal timing, bone acquisition, and risk of fracture throughout life. *Endocr Rev.* 2014;35(5):820−847.
5. Hembree WC, Cohen-Kettenis P, Delemarre-van de Waal HA, et al. Endocrine treatment of transsexual persons: an endocrine society clinical practice guideline. *J Clin Endocrinol Metab.* 2009;94(9):3132−3154.
6. Forwood MR. Primer on the Metabolic Bone Diseases and Disorders of Mineral Metabolism. In: Rosen CJ, ed. 8th ed. Wiley-Blackwell; 2013:149−155.
7. Gilsanz V, Chalfant J, Kalkwarf H, et al. Age at onset of puberty predicts bone mass in young adulthood. *J Pediatr.* 2011;158(1):100−105, 105 e101-102.
8. Finkelstein JS, Klibanski A, Neer RM. A longitudinal evaluation of bone mineral density in adult men with histories of delayed puberty. *J Clin Endocrinol Metab.* 1996;81(3): 1152−1155.
9. Finkelstein JS, Neer RM, Biller BM, Crawford JD, Klibanski A. Osteopenia in men with a history of delayed puberty. *N Engl J Med.* 1992;326(9):600−604.
10. Kindblom JM, Lorentzon M, Norjavaara E, et al. Pubertal timing predicts previous fractures and BMD in young adult men: the GOOD study. *J Bone Miner Res.* 2006;21(5): 790−795.
11. Kuh D, Muthuri SG, Moore A, et al. Pubertal timing and bone phenotype in early old age: findings from a British birth cohort study. *Int J Epidemiol.* 2016;45(4): 1113−1124.
12. Bertelloni S, Baroncelli GI, Ferdeghini M, Menchini-Fabris F, Saggese G. Final height, gonadal function and bone mineral density of adolescent males with central precocious puberty after therapy with gonadotropin-releasing hormone analogues. *Eur J Pediatr.* 2000;159(5):369−374.
13. Yap F, Hogler W, Briody J, Moore B, Howman-Giles R, Cowell CT. The skeletal phenotype of men with previous constitutional delay of puberty. *J Clin Endocrinol Metab.* 2004;89(9):4306−4311.
14. Zhu J, Chan YM. Adult consequences of self-limited delayed puberty. *Pediatrics.* 2017;139(6).

15. Guaraldi F, Beccuti G, Gori D, Ghizzoni L. Management of endocrine disease: long-term outcomes of the treatment of central precocious puberty. *Eur J Endocrinol.* 2016;174(3): R79–R87.

16. Haraldsen IR, Haug E, Falch J, Egeland T, Opjordsmoen S. Cross-sex pattern of bone mineral density in early onset gender identity disorder. *Horm Behav.* 2007;52(3): 334–343.

17. Van Caenegem E, Taes Y, Wierckx K, et al. Low bone mass is prevalent in male-to-female transsexual persons before the start of cross-sex hormonal therapy and gonadectomy. *Bone.* 2013;54(1):92–97.

18. Klink D, Caris M, Heijboer A, van Trotsenburg M, Rotteveel J. Bone mass in young adulthood following gonadotropin-releasing hormone analog treatment and cross-sex hormone treatment in adolescents with gender dysphoria. *J Clin Endocrinol Metab.* 2015;100(2): E270–E275.

19. Vlot MC, Klink DT, den Heijer M, Blankenstein MA, Rotteveel J, Heijboer AC. Effect of pubertal suppression and cross-sex hormone therapy on bone turnover markers and bone mineral apparent density (BMAD) in transgender adolescents. *Bone.* 2016;95:11–19.

20. Cohen-Kettenis PT, Schagen SE, Steensma TD, de Vries AL, Delemarre-van de Waal HA. Puberty suppression in a gender-dysphoric adolescent: a 22-year follow-up. *Arch Sex Behav.* 2011;40(4):843–847.

21. Sisk CL, Zehr JL. Pubertal hormones organize the adolescent brain and behavior. *Front Neuroendocrinol.* 2005; 26(3–4):163–174.

22. Hough D, Bellingham M, Haraldsen IRH, et al. Spatial memory is impaired by peripubertal GnRH agonist treatment and testosterone replacement in sheep. *Psychoneuroendocrinology.* 2017;75:173–182.

23. Hough D, Bellingham M, Haraldsen IR, et al. A reduction in long-term spatial memory persists after discontinuation of peripubertal GnRH agonist treatment in sheep. *Psychoneuroendocrinology.* 2017;77:1–8.

24. Wojniusz S, Callens N, Sutterlin S, et al. Cognitive, emotional, and psychosocial functioning of girls treated with pharmacological puberty blockage for idiopathic central precocious puberty. *Front Psychol.* 2016;7:1053.

25. Grigorova M, Sherwin BB, Tulandi T. Effects of treatment with leuprolide acetate depot on working memory and executive functions in young premenopausal women. *Psychoneuroendocrinology.* 2006;31(8): 935–947.

26. Schneider MA, Spritzer PM, Soll BMB, et al. Brain maturation, cognition and voice pattern in a gender dysphoria case under pubertal suppression. *Front Hum Neurosci.* 2017;11:528.

27. Staphorsius AS, Kreukels BP, Cohen-Kettenis PT, et al. Puberty suppression and executive functioning: an fMRI-study in adolescents with gender dysphoria. *Psychoneuroendocrinology.* 2015;56:190–199.

28. Lazar L, Meyerovitch J, de Vries L, Phillip M, Lebenthal Y. Treated and untreated women with idiopathic precocious puberty: long-term follow-up and reproductive outcome between the third and fifth decades. *Clin Endocrinol (Oxf).* 2014;80(4):570–576.

29. Long CJ, Ginsberg JP, Kolon TF. Fertility preservation in children and adolescents with cancer. *Urology.* 2016;91: 190–196.

30. Wallace WH, Kelsey TW, Anderson RA. Fertility preservation in pre-pubertal girls with cancer: the role of ovarian tissue cryopreservation. *Fertil Steril.* 2016; 105(1):6–12.

31. De Roo C, Tilleman K, T'Sjoen G, De Sutter P. Fertility options in transgender people. *Int Rev Psychiatry.* 2016;28(1): 112–119.

32. Aguiar AL, Couto-Silva AC, Vicente EJ, Freitas IC, Cruz T, Adan L. Weight evolution in girls treated for idiopathic central precocious puberty with GnRH analogues. *J Pediatr Endocrinol Metab.* 2006;19(11):1327–1334.

33. Magiakou MA, Manousaki D, Papadaki M, et al. The efficacy and safety of gonadotropin-releasing hormone analog treatment in childhood and adolescence: a single center, long-term follow-up study. *J Clin Endocrinol Metab.* 2010;95(1):109–117.

34. Schagen SE, Cohen-Kettenis PT, Delemarre-van de Waal HA, Hannema SE. Efficacy and safety of gonadotropin-releasing hormone agonist treatment to suppress puberty in gender dysphoric adolescents. *J Sex Med.* 2016;13(7):1125–1132.

CHAPTER 8

Surgical Side Effects of GnRHa

LOREN S. SCHECHTER, MD, FACS • REBECCA B. SCHECHTER, MD

INTRODUCTION

Gender confirmation surgery can be an important and final step in allowing transgender individuals to become the people they know themselves to be. Not all individuals with gender dysphoria desire surgical therapy, but for those who do, surgery has been shown to be an effective method to alleviate their symptoms and improve their quality of life.[1-8]

Gender confirmation surgery in individuals whose endogenous puberty has been halted with the use of gonadotrophin-releasing hormone agonists (GnRHa) presents several unique considerations. First, the lack of secondary sexual characteristics resulting from GnRHa use may diminish the need for ancillary procedures to feminize or masculinize transgender individuals. Second, the lack of penile growth associated with puberty may limit the applicability of traditional surgical techniques for gender-confirming vaginoplasty. Third, the effect, if any, of GnRHa on other gender-confirming procedures has not been studied. Here we provide an overview of gender confirmation surgeries and the potential advantages and challenges in performing these procedures in individuals treated with GnRHa.

GOALS OF SURGERY

As described in the *The Standards of Care* (WPATH, SOC 7), the overall goal of treatment for transgender individuals is to maximize health, well-being, and fulfillment.[9] Toward this end, gender confirmation surgery can provide the appropriate physical morphology and alleviate the extreme psychological discomfort that many patients experience.[2-4,7,8] Furthermore, as discussed by Meyer in 2001[10] and Cohen-Kettenis and Kuiper in 1984,[11] adjusting the mind to the body is not an effective treatment, while adjusting the body to the mind is the best way to assist severely gender dysphoric persons.

The goal of vaginoplasty is to create a natural-appearing vagina and mons pubis[12] that are sensate and functional. This includes the creation of feminine-appearing labia majora and minora, construction of a sensate neoclitoris, and development of adequate vaginal depth and introital width for intercourse. Additional appealing aspects include a smooth, graded, and contiguous appearance to the labia majora, a moist appearance to the labia minora simulating the vestibular lining in cis-females, clitoral hooding, and lubrication for intercourse. Not all surgical techniques can meet each of these goals, and some individuals may require staged procedures to achieve their surgical goals.

In addition to vaginoplasty, several ancillary procedures are available to transwomen. The overall goal of such surgeries is to aid with feminization of the face, breasts, and body as well as to help alleviate gender dysphoria. These procedures include breast augmentation, reduction thyroid chondroplasty ("tracheal shave"), facial feminization, and body contouring. These procedures can be performed independently from, and either prior to or following genital surgery. The order of surgical procedures depends largely on the aims of the individual.

In transmen, chest surgery is commonly performed, often prior to genital surgery. Gender dysphoria related to breast tissue is often reported, and chest surgery can help alleviate physical and mental discomfort. The goals of chest surgery include aesthetic contouring of the chest by removal of breast tissue and excess skin, reduction and repositioning of the nipple—areola complex when necessary, release of the inframammary crease, liposuction of the chest (if necessary), and, when possible, minimization of chest scars and preservation of nipple sensitivity.[13]

The main options for genital surgery in transmen include metoidioplasty or phalloplasty. The choice for surgery depends on the needs and goals of the individual. Metoidioplasty entails lengthening of the virilized clitoris. It can be performed with urethral lengthening, thereby allowing for urination while standing. However, as metoidioplasty creates a small phallus (typically 5–9 cm in length), penetrative sexual intercourse is typically not possible. Phalloplasty represents the most complete genitoperineal transformation. As outlined by Professor Stan Monstrey, an ideal phallic reconstruction should result in an aesthetic phallus with both tactile and erogenous sensation, the ability to void while standing, minimal morbidity of the surgical intervention and donor site, an aesthetic scrotum, and the ability to experience sexual satisfaction postoperatively.[14]

While the goals of surgery in individuals treated with GnRHa may be similar to those individuals who did not undergo pubertal suppression, the procedures performed to alleviate gender dysphoria may, in some cases, require modification.

TIMING OF SURGERY

One benefit of GnRHa therapy is that by suspending the development of secondary sexual characteristics, individuals have time to explore their gender identity. This is especially important because not all individuals who experience dysphoria ultimately request surgical therapies. For individuals with persistent gender dysphoria who request surgery and are appropriate surgical candidates, the SOC recommends that genital surgery should not be carried out until (1) patients reach the legal age of majority to give consent for medical procedures in a given country and (2) patients have lived continuously for at least 12 months in the gender role that is congruent with their gender identity.[9] The SOC also continues that the age threshold should be seen as a minimum criterion, but it should not be viewed as an indication for intervention. The author (LSS) has performed vaginoplasty surgery on individuals at the age of 17 years, following close consultation with the patient, their family, and their medical and mental health professionals.

Chest surgery in transmen and other ancillary procedures can be carried out earlier than the legal age of majority. In the authors' experience, chest surgery at the age of 17 years is quite common, often following graduation from high school and prior to entering college or the workforce. These cases require careful consideration with the individual, guardian, and entire healthcare team.

In the authors' experience, it is often helpful to pursue certain gender-confirming surgical procedures between major life changes. For example, the transition between high school and college or work can be a good period to pursue chest surgery in transgender adolescents. This allows individuals to start "anew" in the next stage of their life. Furthermore, the support of

friends and family cannot be underestimated. Not only is guardian approval necessary in the case of minors but also, in general, a strong support system is correlated with positive postoperative functioning.[15] The healthcare team should make every effort to work with individuals and their families to ensure a safe and supportive environment prior to pursing surgery.

SURGICAL CONSIDERATIONS FOR INDIVIDUALS ON GnRHa
Surgery for Transwomen on Gonadotrophin-Releasing Hormone Agonists
Vaginoplasty

Many transwomen undergo vaginoplasty to help alleviate dysphoria and improve their quality of life. The surgical options for vaginoplasty consist of one of three approaches: penile disassembly and inversion vaginoplasty, intestinal vaginoplasty, or nongenital flaps/grafts (Fig. 8.1). In general, most centers perform primary vaginoplasty with the penile disassembly and inversion vaginoplasty technique using an anteriorly based penile skin flap combined with a scrotal skin graft. If inadequate penoscrotal tissue is available, full-thickness skin grafts may be harvested from additional sites such as the lower abdomen, flanks, and gluteal folds. However, these sites require incisions in anatomic locations remote from the genitalia. Additionally, if insufficient donor-site tissue is present, tissue expansion may be used to recruit skin from these

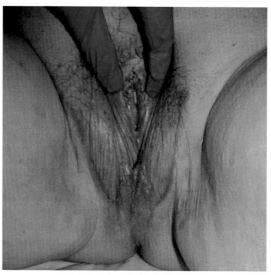

FIG. 8.1 Vaginoplasty.

areas. Tissue expansion entails the subcutaneous placement of a balloon-like device followed by serial instillation of saline on an outpatient basis.

Intestinal vaginoplasty is an alternative to the inversion vaginoplasty technique. Intestinal vaginoplasty is typically reserved for revision cases, but it may be employed as a first-line surgical therapy for those individuals with insufficient penoscrotal tissue. The advantage of intestinal vaginoplasty is the creation of a vascularized 12- to 15-cm vagina with a mucus-secreting, moist lining. The intestinal approach may lessen the requirements for both postoperative vaginal dilation as well as the need for lubrication during intercourse. However, the drawbacks of intestinal vaginoplasty include the need for an intraabdominal operation with a bowel anastomosis and the potential for excess neovaginal secretions with a malodorous discharge.

Due to their soft tissue bulk, nongenital flaps are typically considered for reconstruction following oncologic resections, traumatic repair, or reconstruction following infection. Alternatively, some individuals undergoing vaginoplasty for gender dysphoria do not contemplate vaginal intercourse. Sometimes referred to as a "zero-depth" procedure, this method is used to construct external genitalia (mons pubis, labia majora, labia minora and vestibular lining, and clitoris) without a vaginal canal. While construction of a vaginal canal is possible at a later date, the surgical risks (rectal/urethral/bladder injury) are higher. The zero-depth technique is typically requested by older, non–sexually active individuals or for those individuals deemed at high risk for the traditional vaginoplasty approach. High-risk individuals include those who have undergone previous surgery (i.e., prostatectomy) or radiation to the pelvis/perineum.

In adolescents on GnRHa, the lack of penile length and scrotal volume may limit the utility of penile inversion vaginoplasty, as the neovagina may not have adequate depth. As discussed previously, alternative skin graft donor sites, tissue expansion, or, in select cases, intestinal vaginoplasty may be a first-line therapy. Nongenital flaps/grafts may also be considered, but there is limited experience in the transgender population.

Some individuals may undergo an orchiectomy as an independent procedure prior to vaginoplasty. Because orchiectomy results in permanent infertility, careful consideration is required. Following orchiectomy, GnRHa are no longer needed. If orchiectomy alone is pursued, an incision at the penoscrotal junction is preferred to an inguinal approach. The penoscrotal incision allows access to both the right and left testicles and spermatic cords while preserving the vascular supply to the penile flap, should later vaginoplasty be requested. Although beyond the scope of this chapter, fertility preservation should be discussed prior to sterilizing procedures.

Feminizing procedures

Transwomen may also request surgical procedures to aid with feminization of the face, breast, and body. These procedures include breast augmentation, facial feminization (a constellation of procedures to remove secondary sexual characteristics of the face such as frontal bone reduction, browlift, hairline advancement, rhinoplasty, genioplasty, and mandibular reduction), reduction thyroid chondroplasty ("tracheal shave"), body contouring, and voice surgery.

Breast development in prenatal life is independent of sex hormones and is, therefore, identical in cis-males and cis-females.[16] During embryonic development, breast buds composed of networks of tubules develop from the ectoderm. In cis-females, these tubules will eventually become mature milk ducts. Until puberty, the tubule networks of the breast buds are quiescent. At puberty, breast development diverges in cis-men and cis-women. In cis-females, estrogen and progestins, in conjunction with growth hormone and insulin-like growth factor-1, result in growth and maturation of the tubules into the ductal system of the breasts. Estrogens are generally believed to induce breast proliferation, whereas progestins result in differentiation.[17] Progestins are not thought to have a significant role in breast volume.[18] In contrast, in cis-male puberty, androgens (testosterone and dihydrotestosterone) increase about 10-fold higher compared to cis-females, and estrogen is about 10-fold lower compared to cis-females. The high levels of androgens strongly inhibit the action of estrogen in the breast at puberty, resulting in the lack of breast development in cis-men.

In transwomen, some breast growth occurs with suppression of androgens (GnRHa or spironolactone) and supplementation with estrogens. Breast size typically begins to increase 2–3 months after the start of hormone therapy. Initially, tender breast buds begin to form and breast growth progresses over 2 years.[17,19] Because growth takes place over a period of time, the *SOC* recommends hormone therapy for at least 1 year prior to breast augmentation.[9] However, the response to hormone therapy varies among individuals. Generally, on resolution of breast tenderness, additional clinically significant breast growth is unlikely.

Anatomic differences between the cis-male and cis-female chest are relevant as to implant selection, incision choice, and pocket location.[20] The postpubertal cis-male chest is not only wider than the cis-female chest, but the pectoralis major muscle is usually more robust. Furthermore, the postpubertal cis-male areola is both smaller and more lateral compared to the cis-female areola. However, some of the anatomic issues related to a postpubertal masculinized chest may not be relevant to transwomen treated with GnRHa who have undergone pubertal suppression. Although this issue has not been evaluated in a formal way, transwomen treated with GnRHa may have less masculinized chest physiques. This may result in essentially similar surgical techniques for augmentation mammaplasty in these transwomen as compared to cis females.

Breast implants may be placed in either a subglandular or subpectoral pocket (Fig. 8.2). The decision depends on clinical characteristics including the degree of breast growth in response to hormonal therapy. Subglandular implants may be more palpable and may have higher rates of capsular contracture due to less soft-tissue coverage overlying the implant. However, subpectoral implants may be more prone to displacement and deformities due to the activity of the overlying pectoralis major muscle. Overall, the subpectoral position remains the most common pocket location.

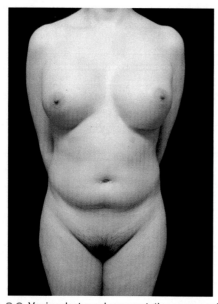

FIG. 8.2 Vaginoplasty and augmentation mammaplasty.

Other feminizing procedures

A variety of characteristics have been identified as male and are often associated with the forehead, nose, malar region, mandible, and thyroid cartilage. These include more pronounced supraorbital bossing in the postpubertal cis-male and a more continuous forehead curvature in the cis-female.[21] The malar region is also more prominent in the cis-female, and the cis-female nose tends to be smaller, with a less acute glabellar angle than the postpubertal cis-male.[21,22] In addition, qualitative and quantitative differences in the skin, subcutaneous tissue, and hair also exist.[23] These differences develop during puberty due to the effects of testosterone. One benefit of using GnRHa in transgender adolescents may be the diminished need for these feminizing procedures. The prevention of stigmatizing secondary sexual characteristics of the face may allow for easier transition to desired gender roles. Furthermore, halting puberty with GnRHa stops the deepening of the voice associated with puberty. This may also decrease the need for voice therapy and surgery in transwomen, both of which may have limited efficacy.[24,25]

Surgery for Transmen on GnRHa

Surgical options for transmen include genital surgery as well as chest surgery. Chest surgery is frequently performed prior to genital surgery and is often the only surgery requested.

Chest surgery

Chest-wall contouring is an important, early surgical step for transmen and may help facilitate their transition. The goals of chest surgery include the aesthetic contouring of the chest by removal of breast tissue and excess skin, reduction and repositioning of the nipple—areola complex when necessary, release of the inframammary crease, liposuction of the chest (if necessary), and, when possible, minimization of chest scars and preservation of nipple sensitivity.[13] In general, chest surgery in transmen can present an aesthetic challenge due to breast volume, breast ptosis, nipple—areola size and position, degree of skin excess, and potential loss of skin elasticity. Breast binding, commonly performed by transmen, may lead to the loss of skin elasticity, thereby necessitating significant amounts of skin removal.

Several surgical methods are utilized, and the choice of technique depends on the skin quality and elasticity, the degree of breast ptosis, and the position of the nipple—areola complex.[13] In addition, preservation of subcutaneous fat on the mastectomy skin flaps, preservation of the pectoralis and serratus fascia, release of the inframammary crease and sternal attachments, and contouring of the lateral chest wall are also important components of chest surgery and chest wall contouring. Preoperative breast imaging (i.e., ultrasound or mammogram) is often performed in older patients, depending on personal and family history, but is generally not necessary in the adolescent population.

Transgender adolescents who initiated GnRHa at Tanner II/II are more likely to have small, nonptotic breasts. In such cases, periareolar incisions ("limited incision") may be adequate to remove the breast tissue. A small amount of tissue is left beneath the nipple—areola to preserve viability (Fig. 8.3A and B). In these cases, nipple reduction and repositioning may not be necessary. This is in contrast to transmen who have larger breasts and require skin removal and/or nipple—areolar reduction and relocation. These procedures include the circumareolar ("pursestring" or "keyhole") +/− vertical/lateral skin incisions with free nipple—areola grafts or transverse inframammary crease incisions ("double incision") with free nipple—areola grafts (Fig. 8.4A and B). In these cases, nipple reduction is commonly employed, often in conjunction with free nipple—areola grafts. In addition, liposuction is frequently used for discontiguous undermining of the inframammary crease and contouring of the lateral and lower chest wall/upper abdomen.

Masculinizing genital surgery

The goal of genital surgery in transgender men depends on the goals of the individual. Surgery may range from simple ("clitoral") release, metoidioplasty with urethral lengthening in order to allow for voiding while standing, to a phalloplasty, capable of sexual penetration.[26]

Metoidioplasty, described in 1996 by Hage, is a less complicated alternative to phalloplasty[27] (Fig. 8.5). The procedure entails lengthening of the hormonally hypertrophied clitoris by release of the ventral chordae, and, when indicated, the suspensory ligament, and the lengthening of the female urethra. Sexual penetration is generally not possible following metoidioplasty, as the constructed phallus is typically 5—9 cm in length and does not allow placement of an implantable penile prosthesis. However, genital sensation is typically maintained and erection of the microphallus is often possible.

Not all individuals request removal of the internal genitalia. However, for those individuals requesting vaginectomy (more aptly colpectomy and colpocleisis) or who are reluctant or refuse ongoing surveillance of the internal genitalia (i.e., routine pap smears), hysterectomy is recommended. Discussions regarding fertility preservation should be undertaken. Most often, individuals requesting "bottom surgery" choose to undergo hysterectomy (and oophorectomy). In these cases, the hysterectomy and oophorectomy are performed at least 2—3 months prior to the metoidioplasty. The metoidioplasty procedure often involves

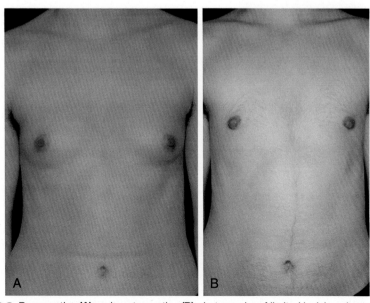

FIG. 8.3 Preoperative **(A)** and postoperative **(B)** photographs of limited incision chest surgery.

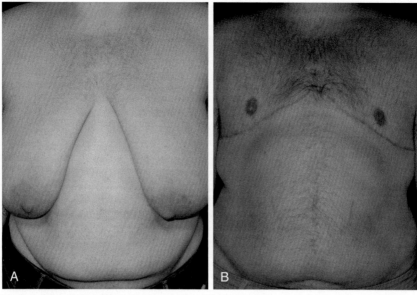

FIG. 8.4 Preoperative **(A)** and postoperative **(B)** photographs of double incision chest surgery.

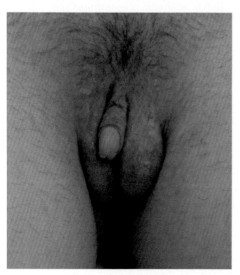

FIG. 8.5 Metoidioplasty.

concomitant removal and closure of the vagina. While often referred to as a "vaginectomy," the procedure is more aptly defined as colpectomy and colpocleisis.[28] In the procedure, a portion of the vagina, incorporating the muscularis layer of the anterior vaginal wall may be used as a flap to reconstruct the proximal portion of the neourethra.[29] The clitoral shaft is degloved and may be further released by detaching

the suspensory ligament from the pubic bone. On the ventral aspect of the clitoris, the urethral plate is divided, allowing straightening and lengthening of the clitoris.[28] Additional lengthening of the urethra is performed with flaps developed from the labia minora.

Scrotoplasty, or creation of a neoscrotum, can be constructed with bilateral labia majora flaps. Testicular implants are typically placed at a secondary surgical procedure so as to reduce the risk of infection and urethral complications.

Phalloplasty, or creation of a functional penis, represents the most complete genital transformation for transgender men (Fig. 8.6A and B). Phalloplasty requires the use of either pedicled flaps (vascularized tissue) or free flaps. Pedicle flaps transfer tissue, typically from the thigh, groin, or lower abdomen to construct the penis, while free flaps involve the microsurgical transfer of tissue from a remote location. Similar to metoidioplasty, hysterectomy and oophorectomy, when desired, are generally performed at least 2—3 months prior to phalloplasty.

The most common technique for penile construction is the radial forearm free flap. This procedure transfers tissue, including blood vessels and nerves, from the forearm to construct the penis and urethra. This flap allows single-stage reconstruction of the urethra as well as a sensate phallus. Potential drawbacks of this technique include the visibility of the donor site on the forearm and the need for microsurgical

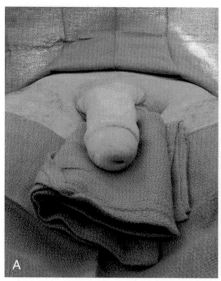 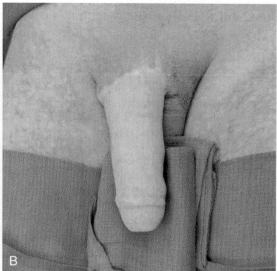

FIG. 8.6 **(A** and **B)** Phalloplasty.

skills. The anterolateral thigh flap is another technique for penile construction. Similar to the forearm technique, tissue, including nerves, may be transferred from the thigh to construct the penis. Depending on the individual's distribution of subcutaneous fat, a second flap may be required for urethral reconstruction. For both the forearm and thigh techniques, the urethra is formed by a skin-lined tube. As such, preoperative electrolysis may be required for depilation (hair removal) of the elongated urethra. Additionally, skin grafting of the donor site (thigh or forearm) is required.

Additional phalloplasty techniques include the use of tissue from the back, known as the musculocutaneous latissimus dorsi flap. One notable downside of this flap is the lack of a sensory nerve to the tissue that will be used to construct the phallus. Additionally, the flap is often excessively bulky.

Following phalloplasty, testicular implants and penile prostheses can be placed at a secondary procedure, allowing for penetrative intercourse. While testicular implants may be placed several months following the phalloplasty, the penile prosthesis is typically placed 9−12 months after the initial procedure so as to allow the phallus to achieve protective sensation through reinnervation.

The effect of GnRHa on transmen who pursue metoidioplasty or phalloplasty is not well understood. In contrast to transwomen on GnRHa who desire penile inversion vaginoplasty, virilization of the clitoris and labia minora may result from exogenous testosterone. As such, the amount of available genital tissue may be less of a concern for transmen desiring "bottom surgery."

AREAS OF UNCERTAINTY

From a surgical standpoint, one advantage of pubertal suppression may be a lessened need/desire for invasive surgical procedures (i.e., limited-incision chest surgery as opposed to double-incision chest surgery with free nipple grafts) or even the ability to forego certain procedures (i.e., facial feminization). However, one potential drawback is the need to develop alternate surgical techniques for genital reconstruction, especially in transwomen. If, as a result of pubertal suppression, full penile length is not realized, alternate methodologies (i.e., intestinal vaginoplasty, tissue expansion, remote flaps/grafts) may be required in order to construct a functional vagina.

The effect of GnRHa on gender-confirming surgical procedures is an emerging area. While the benefits of pubertal suppression for procedures such as chest surgery in transmen are better understood, the impact of pubertal suppression on genital surgery is evolving based on a limited number of cases. Several important questions require ongoing study and include: what is the best vaginoplasty technique for transgender youth on GnRHa? Are augmentation mammaplasty techniques and implant size affected by the use of GnRHa? Are facial feminization procedures necessary? Is limited-incision chest surgery adequate for masculinizing the chest wall? Do GnRHa affect the techniques used for metoidioplasty or phalloplasty?

CONCLUSION

GnRHa provide transgender youth an excellent opportunity to explore their gender identity by suspending the progression of puberty. For those who go on to pursue gender confirmation procedures, GnRHa provide several potential benefits including diminished need for facial feminization procedures and less invasive mastectomy techniques such as "limited incision" chest surgery. Therapy with GnRHa also presents challenges to gender confirmation surgeons when determining the most effective technique for vaginoplasty. Furthermore, many topics require additional study, such as the effect of GnRHa on masculinizing genital surgery. With increased awareness, advocacy, and access to medical care, the use of GnRHa in youth with gender dysphoria is likely to increase. As such, exploring how to best provide surgical care for appropriate individuals will continue to evolve.

REFERENCES

1. Monstrey S, Hoebeke P, Dhont M, et al. Surgical therapy in transsexual patients: a multi-disciplinary approach. *Acta Chir Belg.* 2001;101(5):200−209.
2. Mate-Kole C, Freschi M, Robin A. A controlled study of psychological and social change after surgical gender reassignment in selected male transsexuals. *Br J Psychiatry.* August 1990;157:261−264.
3. Imbimbo C, Verze P, Palmieri A, et al. A report from a single institute's 14-year experience in treatment of male-to-female transsexuals. *J Sex Med.* 2009;6(10):2736−2745.
4. Weyers S, Elaut E, De Sutter P, et al. Long-term assessment of the physical, mental, and sexual health among transsexual women. *J Sex Med.* 2009;6(3):752−760.
5. Vujovic S, Popovic S, Sbutega-Milosevic G, Djordjevic M, Gooren L. Transsexualism in Serbia: a twenty-year follow-up study. *J Sex Med.* 2009;6(4):1018−1023.
6. Kockott G, Fahrner EM. Transsexuals who have not undergone surgery: a follow-up study. *Arch Sex Behav.* 1987;16(6):511−522.
7. Johansson A, Sundbom E, Hojerback T, Bodlund O. A five-year follow-up study of Swedish adults with gender identity disorder. *Arch Sex Behav.* 2010;39(6):1429−1437.
8. Cohen-Kettenis P, Pfafflin F. *Transgenderism and Intersexuality in Children and Adolescence: Making Choices.* Thousand Oaks, CA: Sage; 2003.
9. World Professional Association for Transgender Health Standards of Care. https://s3.amazonaws.com/amo_hub_content/Association140/files/Standards%20of%20Care%20V7%20-%202011%20WPATH%20(2)(1).pdf; 2012.
10. Meyer IH. Why lesbian, gay, bisexual, and transgender public health? *Am J Public Health.* 2001;91(6):856−859.
11. Cohen-Kettenis P, Kuiper B. Transseksualiteit en psychotherapie. *Tijdschr Voor Psychother.* 1984;3:153.
12. Seitz IA, Wu C, Retzlaff K, Zachary L. Measurements and aesthetics of the mons pubis in normal weight females. *Plast Reconstr Surg.* 2010;126(1):46e−48e.
13. Monstrey S, Selvaggi G, Ceulemans P, et al. Chest-wall contouring surgery in female-to-male transsexuals: a new algorithm. *Plast Reconstr Surg.* 2008;121(3):849−859.
14. Monstrey S, Hoebeke P, Selvaggi G, et al. Penile reconstruction: is the radial forearm flap really the standard technique? *Plast Reconstr Surg.* 2009;124(2):510−518.
15. Eldh J, Berg A, Gustafsson M. Long-term follow up after sex reassignment surgery. *Scand J Plast Reconstr Surg Hand Surg.* 1997;31(1):39−45.
16. Javed A, Lteif A. Development of the human breast. *Semin Plast Surg.* 2013;27(1):5−12.
17. Wierckx K, Gooren L, T'Sjoen G. Clinical review: breast development in trans women receiving cross-sex hormones. *J Sex Med.* 2014;11(5):1240−1247.
18. Hembree WC, Cohen-Kettenis P, Delemarre-van de Waal HA, et al. Endocrine treatment of transsexual persons: an endocrine society clinical practice guideline. *J Clin Endocrinol Metab.* 2009;94(9):3132−3154.
19. Dahl M, Feldman J, Goldberg J, et al. Physial aspects of transgender endocrine therapy. *Int J Transgend.* 2006;9(3/4):111−134.
20. Kanhai RC, Hage JJ, Asscheman H, Mulder JW. Augmentation mammaplasty in male-to-female transsexuals. *Plast Reconstr Surg.* 1999;104(2):542−549. discussion 550−541.
21. Ousterhout DK. Feminization of the forehead: contour changing to improve female aesthetics. *Plast Reconstr Surg.* 1987;79(5):701−713.
22. Hage JJ, Vossen M, Becking AG. Rhinoplasty as part of gender-confirming surgery in male transsexuals: basic considerations and clinical experience. *Ann Plast Surg.* 1997;39(3):266−271.
23. Hage JJ, Becking AG, de Graaf FH, Tuinzing DB. Gender-confirming facial surgery: considerations on the masculinity and femininity of faces. *Plast Reconstr Surg.* 1997;99(7):1799−1807.
24. Lechien JR, Delvaux V, Huet K, et al. [Transgender voice and communication treatment: review of the literature]. *Rev Laryngol Otol Rhinol Bord.* 2014;135(2):97−103.
25. McNeill EJ. Management of the transgender voice. *J Laryngol Otol.* 2006;120(7):521−523.
26. Hage JJ, van Turnhout AA, Dekker JJ, Karim RB. Saving labium minus skin to treat possible urethral stenosis in female-to-male transsexuals. *Ann Plast Surg.* 2006;56(4):456−459.

27. Hage JJ. Metaidoioplasty: an alternative phalloplasty technique in transsexuals. *Plast Reconstr Surg.* 1996;97(1): 161−167.

28. Djordjevic ML, Bizic M, Stanojevic D, et al. Urethral Lengthening in metoidioplasty (female-to-male sex reassignment surgery) by combined buccal mucosa graft and labia minora flap. *Urology.* 2009;74(2):349−353.

29. Hage JJ, Torenbeek R, Bouman FG, Bloem JJ. The anatomic basis of the anterior vaginal flap used for neourethra construction in female-to-male transsexuals. *Plast Reconstr Surg.* 1993;92(1):102−108. discussion 109.

CHAPTER 9

Fertility Preservation: Considerations for Gender-Diverse Youth

ANNA VALENTINE, MD • AMY C. TISHELMAN, PHD • LEENA NAHATA, MD

With an increasing number of gender-diverse youth seeking medical and surgical gender-affirming care,[1,2] concerns have been raised about implications of these interventions for future fertility.[3] Studies have shown adults with fertility impairment due to a variety of conditions or treatments prescribed in childhood/ adolescence experience distress and regrets about their inability to have biologically related children.[4–7] Given the expanding body of literature in other at-risk pediatric populations (such as oncology), organizations such as The World Professional Association for Transgender Health, Endocrine Society, and the American Society for Reproductive Medicine have published guidelines urging providers to discuss infertility risk and fertility preservation (FP) options with gender-diverse youth and families prior to initiating hormone therapies and surgeries.[3,8,9] Others have called for a general integration of fertility and sexual function counseling into care for at-risk pediatric populations.[10,11] This chapter seeks to describe the potential impact of the three most common hormonal therapies used in gender-diverse youth (gonadotropin-releasing hormone agonists [GnRHa], testosterone, estrogen), outline various FP options based on pubertal stage, review relevant literature with regard to FP utilization in this population, and discuss salient psychological, ethical, and financial considerations. Acknowledging that terminology is continuing to evolve, the terms "gender diverse" or "cis/transgender," and "birth assigned" or "natal" will be used for the purposes of this chapter.

RISK OF INFERTILITY DUE TO HORMONAL THERAPIES

Given the paucity of long-term data among gender-diverse individuals treated with hormonal therapies in childhood/adolescence, infertility risk assessment remains a challenge. Based on clinical experience with adults who have been previously treated with GnRHa for precocious puberty (testicular enlargement prior to 9 years of age in birth-assigned males and breast development before 8 years of age in birth-assigned females), these agents are not known to directly impair fertility. However, GnRHa prevent maturation of gametes and suppress the endogenous hypothalamic–pituitary–gonadal axis, and treatment with GnRHa has been shown to cause a decrease in testicular volumes in birth-assigned males (i.e., sperm-producing cells).[12] Notably, many gender-diverse youth being treated with these agents progress directly to other hormonal therapies (e.g., testosterone, estrogen), and/or surgical interventions that impact reproductive capacity to varying degrees; GnRHa would thus need to be stopped for a period of time prior to pursuing these other therapies in order to complete FP.

Studies on the impact of estrogen therapy on testicular morphology have shown inconsistent results, yet have raised concerns about impact on spermatogenesis.[13] Administration of ethinyl estradiol among transgender females has shown to quickly result in a physiologic decrease in follicle-stimulating hormone along with abnormalities in sperm motility, and to a lesser extent a decrease in luteinizing hormone and lower sperm density profiles measured in semen.[14] Small studies among transgender females undergoing gonadectomy have shown a negative impact of long-term exogenous estrogen on testicular architecture and makeup among many (but not all) individuals, raising concerns about overall impact on fertility.[15,16]

Histological studies show ovarian tissue remains relatively normal after short-term testosterone exposure.[17] After long-term testosterone administration, however, changes may be seen similar to those in polycystic ovarian syndrome (PCOS) including multiple cystic follicles, collagenization, and stromal hyperplasia, suggesting this as a potential mechanism for fertility impairment.[18] Other studies have shown that testosterone accelerates follicular atresia as another potential mechanism for fertility impairment.[19] Interestingly, in another study, over half of transgender male adults had biochemical evidence of PCOS *prior* to initiating any hormone therapy, including about 40% with hyperandrogenism[20]; thus, it is possible that fertility difficulties may be present in some transgender individuals even prior to starting testosterone therapy. That being said, there have been reported pregnancies among transgender males after cessation of testosterone therapy.[21] One study that examined the qualities of transgender males having delivered a neonate showed that over half of them had taken testosterone, and most (88%) had used their own oocytes to achieve pregnancy.[21] Health outcomes of those offspring have not been examined.

Despite the limited evidence and lack of consensus about long-term effects of hormonal therapies on fertility, published guidelines and authors of contemporary studies state that conversations about potential risk and FP options should begin early in the course of evaluation and treatment and continue on an ongoing basis.[8,22] Notably, there is significant variation in timing of GnRHa initiation among gender-diverse youth, with some starting at Tanner stage 2 and others starting at older ages/later stages in puberty.[23] This is particularly important when considering fertility, as postpubertal adolescents may have access to FP options that are established, whereas those who present in Tanner stage 2 requesting hormone therapy (e.g., GnRHa) may never achieve "natal" puberty and therefore have fewer FP options.[24]

FERTILITY PRESERVATION OPTIONS IN BIRTH-ASSIGNED MALES

Sperm cryopreservation is an established and effective FP option for birth-assigned males who have reached at least Tanner stage 2–3 in puberty.[24] The least invasive and most cost-effective option is to collect semen for cryopreservation from an ejaculated sample, and identify a cryopreservation facility that can process and store the sample long term. Studies have shown that this method can be successful in youth as young as 13 years.[25] While some adolescents may be comfortable with this option, others may be sexually inexperienced and/or find this process psychologically difficult due to their gender dysphoria. Studies have shown that cisgender males who are considering sperm banking prior to different types of gonadotoxic

therapies may face challenges due to young age and sexual inexperience, embarrassment, or guilt/shame associated with cultural, religious, or personal beliefs that discourage masturbation.[26–29]

If it is not possible to collect an ejaculated sperm sample, alternative methods including electroejaculation (EEJ), testicular sperm extraction (TESE), or testicular sperm aspiration (TESA) may be considered.[30,31] EEJ is a procedure usually performed under anesthesia, in which a rectal probe is used to deliver a mild electric current to stimulate an ejaculation; the equipment may not be available at every center.[30] In TESE/TESA, the patient undergoes testicular biopsy or needle aspiration of sperm from the testes/epididymis under sedation in the operating room, or with local anesthesia in the office.[32,33] Successful retrieval has been reported among males with testes as small as 6 mL.[34] Of note, these methods may carry a small degree of medical risk and may also have significant expenses associated with anesthesia and employment of a more invasive method, since insurance coverage is often limited.

The previously described sperm preservation techniques are not possible among prepubertal males (or those just starting puberty), as their bodies are not yet producing mature sperm. While there are no FP options that guarantee future viable sperm for use in assisted reproduction, testicular tissue cryopreservation (TTC) is an experimental method being offered at several centers.[35,36] Procedures have been established for extracting tissue from a prepubertal testis in hopes of isolating immature gametes in the form of spermatogonial stem cells (SSCs) to cryopreserve, showing promising results in animal models.[37–39] These SSCs have been kept both in cell suspension and in tissue that includes Sertoli cells.[40] The hope is that the cryopreserved tissue can be combined with tailored media to induce spermatogenesis for eventual in vitro maturation to produce viable sperm to be used in in vitro fertilization/intracytoplasmic sperm injection[39]; however, no live births have yet been reported in humans.

FERTILITY PRESERVATION OPTIONS IN BIRTH-ASSIGNED FEMALES

In birth-assigned females who have experienced menarche, established FP options include embryo cryopreservation and oocyte cryopreservation; the latter is more common in pediatrics, as no sperm donor is needed.[24,41] Ovarian stimulation with oocyte retrieval is performed using a similar approach as in cisgender women undergoing in vitro fertilization procedures; gonadotropin injections are administered for 8—14 days to induce ovulation.[42] Follicles are monitored by transvaginal ultrasound, and oocyte retrieval is then performed transvaginally by needle aspiration under ultrasound guidance. While this method is commonly employed by reproductive endocrinologists and has been successfully performed in adolescents,[42] the injections and method of oocyte retrieval can understandably be challenging for this population and come with the risk of ovarian hyperstimulation syndrome, intraabdominal bleeding, and procedural risks.[41,43]

Prior to initiating ovarian stimulation and oocyte retrieval methods, it is prudent to discuss with patients and families that exogenous testosterone may not render their ovarian tissue incapable of producing oocytes if testosterone is discontinued, as several case reports have been published describing pregnancies in transgender men who have stopped their testosterone therapy.[21] As described above, however, little is known about infertility risk after longstanding testosterone therapy (i.e., initiated in adolescence). In studies looking at fertility outcomes in women with PCOS, who have higher than physiologic levels of circulating testosterone, treatment with ovulation-inducing agents has shown potential for pregnancy in 30%—82%[44]; there are risks associated with using these agents, and it remains unclear whether there would be similar outcomes as seen in PCOS. If considering this pathway for future reproduction, it will be important to discuss that temporarily discontinuing testosterone therapy may lead to a gender presentation less consistent with their gender identity and to encourage these individuals to consider the potential psychological ramifications of pursuing this route.

As with birth-assigned males, the only FP option for prepubertal (premenarchal) birth-assigned females is ovarian tissue cryopreservation (OTC), which is considered experimental.[45] The recommended procedure is a laparoscopic unilateral oophorectomy with cryopreservation of ovarian cortical tissue.[46,47] Contrary to TTC, there have been ~80 human live births reported from cryopreserved ovarian tissue[48,49]; notably, however, only one of these reports has been from tissue extracted from a prepubertal child.[50] Since OTC in prepubertal children often requires removal of a complete ovary, institutional review board (IRB) protocols typically specify that this procedure should only be considered in patients at high risk of developing primary ovarian insufficiency.[45] Thus, given the limited data on impact of testosterone treatment of ovarian function and long-term outcomes of OTC among prepubertal youth,

this procedure may not be appropriate for gender-diverse youth undergoing hormone therapy. However, OTC should be considered in older gender-diverse individuals pursuing any gender-affirming surgeries including gonadectomy.

Of note, the only reported human births from cryopreserved ovarian tissue have occurred after tissue reimplantation into the human body (e.g., after cancer treatment is complete and the patient is cancer free), such that it may be exposed to endogenous gonadotropins and start producing estrogen and progesterone in a cyclical manner.[45] This limits the use of this technology even in oncologic populations, as patients with hematologic malignancies may be at risk for reintroduction of malignancy through reimplantation of ovarian tissue.[51] The ovarian tissue reimplantation method may also be less desirable for some transgender adults as the gonad and potential results of hormonal stimulation are not consistent with their gender identity. With ongoing research efforts, in vitro maturation protocols are being refined to allow for more widespread use of this FP method.[52]

ATTITUDES TOWARD FP AND OTHER PSYCHOLOGICAL CONSIDERATIONS

In spite of these technological advances, FP utilization remains inconsistent, and significant psychosocial challenges exist in pediatric populations. The majority of studies focusing on FP attitudes and uptake in youth have been done in pediatric oncology, as chemotherapy and gonadal radiation have been known to damage gonadal function. Primary findings are as follows: (1) standardizing procedures for counseling about risk and FP options increases FP uptake and improves patient satisfaction[53−56]; (2) 25%—50% of pubertal boys who receive counseling attempt to bank sperm prior to chemotherapy/radiation and FP uptake in other groups (pubertal females, prepubertal males and females) is more variable[57,58]; (3) parental recommendation has an important impact on FP decisions among youth[28]; (4) many adult survivors of childhood cancer report distress about potential infertility and regret missed opportunities for FP.[4,5,59]

Far fewer studies have been conducted examining parenthood goals and fertility-related attitudes among other populations such as gender-diverse individuals. While some studies have shown adults in the LGBTQ community may be less interested in having children and more open to alternate options for parenthood,[60] several other studies have shown that transgender adults frequently express interest in parenting biologically related children and regret not having known about FP options prior to their transition.[61-63] Additionally, recent research among transgender adults has highlighted physical, social, and legal barriers associated with pursuing fertility/parenthood options,[63-65] yet many have succeeded using various methods.[21,66]

Attitudes toward parenthood in transgender youth have been less broadly studied to date, but recent literature has shown that <5% opt for FP when offered prior to initiating gender-affirming hormone therapy.[67,68] The reasons for their reluctance are relatively unexplored, although they are likely multifactorial, and may include factors unique to the individual and family, developmental factors relevant to adolescents in general, and variables germane to the specific circumstances of transgender teens. The most common documented reasons for refusal in a recent study included a preference for adoption or denial of any desire for future children.[67] Less common barriers were cost, discomfort masturbating to produce a semen sample, and having to delay hormonal treatment in order to pursue FP options.[67]

One of the many challenges in conducting research in this population is the lack of appropriate measures. A survey was recently developed to assess FP attitudes and support fertility-related clinical conversations with gender-diverse youth and families.[69] With regard to desire for children, almost all youth and parents said it was important to learn how hormone therapies could impact fertility (most had received information online); just over half of the adolescents indicated a wish to have children; the majority of youth said they would consider adoption.[69] Approximately half of parents reported wanting to learn about FP options and wanting their children to consider FP.[69] Notably, almost half of the youth acknowledged that their feelings about wanting a biological child might change in the future,[69] yet research applying a developmental perspective on parenthood goals in transgender youth is lacking.

Whenever possible, an interdisciplinary model of care may offer the best structure for fertility discussions. A comprehensive evaluation and support from a mental health provider with expertise in gender dysphoria is crucial, particularly given the increased mental health concerns in this population,[23] and potential impact of these conditions on FP decisions. Although outcomes appear to be better among transgender youth supported by peers and families,[70] several articles describe challenges faced by many

transgender children and adolescents, including anxiety, depression, and suicidality.[71,72] Depression and suicidality can impact an adolescent's future expectations, concentration, and attention and even the motivation to engage in complex discussions, as future considerations may seem irrelevant. The lack of acceptance from families, communities, and peers can increase mental health risks in this vulnerable population of youth[60] and could potentially impact attitudes and beliefs about family and parenthood. Autism spectrum symptoms have been found to be elevated in transgender youth seeking hormonal intervention, which can impact thought processes and comprehension of complex issues.[73,74] Therefore, it is critical for counseling regarding fertility issues to take into account an adolescent's state of mind during these important conversations and to have a basic understanding of a youth's sense of safety, family relationships, and trust, which can be more exposed to disruption and high volatility for gender-diverse youth seeking medical interventions than for youth typically cared for in a medical context. Appropriate psychological assessment is warranted prior to counseling to inform the process and allow for a flexible approach individually tailored to the needs of each adolescent and family, and to ensure that adolescents are psychologically able to engage in the process of informed decision-making.[75]

Some research in other clinical realms has addressed best practices in adolescent communication with a clinical team in general, and these can be extrapolated to the context of fertility counseling in transgender youth healthcare. For instance, research indicates that effective communication involves professionals adopting certain behaviors that may enhance rapport, including compassionate responses and avoiding giving the message to a patient of being rushed and unable to devote the necessary time for important conversations.[76] Given the complex nature of fertility counseling with transgender youth, it makes sense for team members to ensure that clinic procedures for fertility counseling are clear, sensitive, and allot enough time for adolescents and their parents to engage in a multiple-session process of careful discussion and reflection.

ETHICAL CONSIDERATIONS

Given the limited data on infertility risk and fertility outcomes after experimental FP procedures, psychological considerations, and financial challenges (described below), ethical dilemmas frequently arise in fertility-related care for gender-diverse youth. Data in cancer suggest that comprehensive discussions should occur surrounding overall risk of infertility, potential psychological stressors of future infertility and the inability to parent genetic offspring, the need for a separate procedure to harvest gonadal tissue, delay of treatment of primary medical concern, and success rates of the proposed technique.[77]

As discussed above, sperm cryopreservation is generally a low-risk FP method compared to other FP options. The most obvious potential risks to consider include those associated with any surgical procedure, including bleeding, infection, and exposure to general anesthesia. Unlike patients with cancer who could have FP procedures coordinated with line placement/other procedures requiring sedation or general anesthesia, transgender youth do not have surgical procedures or sedation as a part of their routine care, thus introducing an added risk of exposure to anesthesia that they would not otherwise have. In addition, since gender-affirming hormone therapy does not necessarily exclude a transgender person's ability to regain fertility potential if gender-affirming therapies are discontinued, risk of infertility needs to be weighed against risk of an FP procedure. General care guidelines established by oncologists have suggested that due to the experimental nature of gonadal tissue cryopreservation, its application should generally only be offered under approved IRB protocols in which a family is fully consented.[78]

Professional guidelines indicate that it is appropriate and important to include adolescents in decision-making about important medical interventions.[79] This may be particularly relevant with transgender youth, who often have preexisting distress related to their bodies, and in particular reproductive anatomy that may be discordant with their identified gender. In some situations, it could be psychologically contraindicated and possibly harmful to require invasive FP interventions without giving youth control over this process. The mature-minor doctrine recognizes that many adolescents are sufficiently mature and able to provide independent informed consent for medical care, accounting for the complexities of decision-making.[79] Research from other arenas of pediatric healthcare suggests that adolescents have the desire to be involved in decision-making.[80] In general, adolescents are able to engage in thoughtful decision-making about their own clinical care, although they may tend to rely more on socioemotional rather than cognitive control systems or, in other words, be

more prone toward impulsive decision-making and short-term thinking than adult counterparts. As the American Academy of Pediatrics (AAP) notes "clinicians should generally advocate for the adolescent's wishes if they represent an ethically acceptable treatment option."[79]

The AAP Committee on Bioethics also outlines the elements of informed consent/assent for medical decision-making, including the provision of full information about treatment and its implication, and practical issues such as an assessment of the factors that may be influencing an adolescent's response.[79] Allotting sufficient time for discussion may also enable parents to explore their own feelings, as well as their child's perspective separate from theirs, facilitating more positive and respectful interactions. In other words, simply providing information regarding the impacts of hormonal treatments on fertility and fertility-sparing options is not sufficient. Fertility discussions may need to occur numerous times, and sometimes with both medical and mental health providers in order to make sure the factual information is sufficiently understood, and to allow time for consideration of options. An adolescent's first response may not reflect their eventual decision, and they should be given enough time for considering short- and long-term goals. This becomes challenging as many youth feel an urgency to begin hormonal interventions and are reticent to take time to weigh options.

It may be helpful to inform youth about the preliminary research indicating that transgender adults sometimes express a desire for biological children.[61–63] However, these discussions should be moderated and balanced with the understanding that healthcare providers should be sensitive to the risk of being perceived as harassing or trying to coerce an unwilling teen. Youth and their parents may not always agree, creating challenges for ultimately coming up with a plan for FP. This discord may make an already tense situation (e.g., in families who are struggling with other aspects of their child's transition) even worse.[81] If enough time is allotted to fertility-related discussions, it should be possible to understand all the differing concerns of individuals in a family, and with counseling, it may be possible to come to a comfortable consensus and plan.[82]

FINANCIAL CONSIDERATIONS

One of the most significant barriers to FP in any population is cost.[83] FP procedures, processing, and storage are poorly covered by insurance in many parts of the

United States.[84] For birth-assigned females, procedures such as oocyte freezing and OTC can cost approximately $5000–20,000, with extra annual fees for continued freezing that average about $300–500 per year. The financial burden tends to be less overall for birth-assigned males if they can provide a sperm sample via masturbation ($500–$1500 up front plus $300–500 per year storage fee), but these individuals can also be faced with larger costs if sperm retrieval via EEJ or biopsy is chosen, running anywhere from $1000 to $16,000 in addition to storage fees.[85] It is important to note that gender-diverse individuals may face additional challenges, as (1) FP procedures cannot be coordinated with other planned procedures (such as biopsies or central line placements occurring in youth with cancer) and (2) gender-related care is poorly covered overall, leading to a higher financial burden for some of these families even without FP added expenses.[23] While costs can be high, it is important to offer these options to families as studies in the pediatric oncology population have shown overall improved satisfaction in care and communication when FP was considered prior to undergoing therapy that could affect future fertility.[54]

FUTURE DIRECTIONS

As current options in FP for gender-diverse youth largely draw upon what is already established in adult medicine as well as what is available for pediatric cancer patients at risk for infertility, more dedicated studies are needed to understand the needs of transgender and other gender diverse populations with regard to FP. Prospective studies on parenthood goals and perceived benefits/barriers to FP could help practitioners provide better, more culturally competent care. While some barriers (physical discomfort with FP methods, financial barriers) are more straightforward, other topics have not been investigated. For example, in a recent study, a large cohort of youth indicated an intention to adopt,[67] yet little is known about the adoption experiences and feasibility of adoption in a political landscape that is changing. Research should examine potential obstacles such as cost of adoption (which may be equivalent to costs associated with FP), and the potential impact of biases toward transgender individuals on adoption success. Further, since preliminary investigation shows more transgender adults are interested in parenting biological children than would be suspected on the basis of rates of youth opting for

fertility-sparing interventions,[61–63,67,68] longitudinal studies are needed to examine perspectives over time. The possibility of decisional regret and ultimate parenthood desires should be systematically examined.

While research in other pediatric populations can inform best practices with transgender youth,[54,58] the concerns of youth with other medical conditions, such as cancer, diverge in important ways from potential concerns of transgender youth. For instance, youth with cancer sometimes have unclear survival prognoses and may have a limited time to consider fertility options prior to the onset of treatment, which are considerations that do not necessarily impact transgender youth. Transgender adolescents may have other considerations that are idiosyncratic to their circumstances as well. As mentioned above, family discord (related to the transition in general)[81] may negatively skew an adolescent's idea of a family and their desire to be a future parent, and mental health conditions such as depression and anxiety[23] can impact perceptions of future parenting goals. High rates of peer victimization and social isolation[60] may potentially impact thinking about future likelihood of intimate partnerships and family goals. These issues do not absolve professionals from responsibilities to engage adolescents in decision-making about fertility but do require further investigation.

CONCLUSIONS

In summary, healthcare providers have a responsibility to provide adequate counsel about infertility risk and FP options to gender-diverse youth and their families prior to initiating any treatments that may impair fertility. An interdisciplinary approach, including both medical and mental health providers, is optimal. Prospective studies are needed to (1) gain a better understanding of parenthood goals at different ages and developmental stages, (2) examine fertility outcomes after hormonal therapies that are initiated in childhood/adolescence, and (3) inform more optimal approaches for fertility counseling for children and adolescents whose sense of urgency to begin medical transition may be prioritized over FP. Further, technological advances are needed to improve cell culture and cryopreservation methods that are currently experimental. Lessons should be learned from research in other populations (such as pediatric oncology), with a commitment to conduct studies in this population and practice evidence-based care.

REFERENCES

1. Spack NP, Edwards-Leeper L, Feldman HA, et al. Children and adolescents with gender identity disorder referred to a pediatric medical center. *Pediatrics*. 2012;129(3):418–425.
2. Aitken M, Steensma TD, Blanchard R, et al. Evidence for an altered sex ratio in clinic-referred adolescents with gender dysphoria. *J Sex Med*. 2015;12(3):756–763.
3. Hembree WC, Cohen-Kettenis PT, Gooren L, et al. Endocrine treatment of gender-dysphoric/gender-incongruent persons: an endocrine society clinical practice guideline. *J Clin Endocrinol Metab*. 2017;102(11):3869–3903.
4. Nilsson J, Jervaeus A, Lampic C, et al. 'Will I be able to have a baby?' Results from online focus group discussions with childhood cancer survivors in Sweden. *Hum Reprod*. 2014; 29(12):2704–2711.
5. Ellis SJ, Wakefield CE, McLoone JK, Robertson EG, Cohn RJ. Fertility concerns among child and adolescent cancer survivors and their parents: a qualitative analysis. *J Psychosoc Oncol*. 2016;34(5):347–362.
6. Canada AL, Schover LR. The psychosocial impact of interrupted childbearing in long-term female cancer survivors. *Psychooncology*. 2012;21(2):134–143.
7. Gorman JR, Su HI, Roberts SC, Dominick SA, Malcarne VL. Experiencing reproductive concerns as a female cancer survivor is associated with depression. *Cancer*. 2015;121(6): 935–942.
8. Coleman E, Bockting W, Botzer M, et al. Standards of care for the health of transsexual, transgender, and gender-nonconforming people, Version 7. *Int J Transgend*. 2012; 13(4):165–232.
9. Ethics Committee of the American Society for Reproductive M. Access to fertility services by transgender persons: an Ethics Committee opinion. *Fertil Steril*. 2015;104(5): 1111–1115.
10. Nahata L, Quinn GP, Tishelman A. A call for fertility and sexual function counseling in pediatrics. *Pediatrics*. 2016; 137(6).
11. Johnson EK, Finlayson C, Rowell EE, et al. Fertility preservation for pediatric patients: current state and future possibilities. *J Urol*. 2017;198.
12. Schagen SE, Cohen-Kettenis PT, Delemarre-van de Waal HA, Hannema SE. Efficacy and safety of gonadotropin-releasing hormone agonist treatment to suppress puberty in gender dysphoric adolescents. *J Sex Med*. 2016;13(7):1125–1132.
13. Schneider F, Kliesch S, Schlatt S, Neuhaus N. Andrology of male-to-female transsexuals: influence of cross-sex hormone therapy on testicular function. *Andrology*. 2017; 5(5):873–880.
14. Lubbert H, Leo-Rossberg I, Hammerstein J. Effects of ethinyl estradiol on semen quality and various hormonal parameters in a eugonadal male. *Fertil Steril*. 1992;58(3): 603–608.
15. Schulze C. Response of the human testis to long-term estrogen treatment: morphology of Sertoli cells, Leydig cells and spermatogonial stem cells. *Cell Tissue Res*. 1988; 251(1):31–43.

16. Thiagaraj D, Gunasegaram R, Loganath A, Peh KL, Kottegoda SR, Ratnam SS. Histopathology of the testes from male transsexuals on oestrogen therapy. *Ann Acad Med Singap*. 1987;16(2):347–348.
17. De Roo C, Lierman S, Tilleman K, et al. Ovarian tissue cryopreservation in female-to-male transgender people: insights into ovarian histology and physiology after prolonged androgen treatment. *Reprod Biomed Online*. 2017; 34(6):557–566.
18. Spinder T, Spijkstra JJ, van den Tweel JG, et al. The effects of long term testosterone administration on pulsatile luteinizing hormone secretion and on ovarian histology in eugonadal female to male transsexual subjects. *J Clin Endocrinol Metab*. 1989;69(1):151–157.
19. Ikeda K, Baba T, Noguchi H, et al. Excessive androgen exposure in female-to-male transsexual persons of reproductive age induces hyperplasia of the ovarian cortex and stroma but not polycystic ovary morphology. *Hum Reprod*. 2013;28(2):453–461.
20. Baba T, Endo T, Honnma H, et al. Association between polycystic ovary syndrome and female-to-male transsexuality. *Hum Reprod*. 2007;22(4):1011–1016.
21. Light AD, Obedin-Maliver J, Sevelius JM, Kerns JL. Transgender men who experienced pregnancy after female-to-male gender transitioning. *Obstet Gynecol*. 2014;124(6): 1120–1127.
22. T'Sjoen G, Van Caenegem E, Wierckx K. Transgenderism and reproduction. *Curr Opin Endocrinol Diabetes Obes*. 2013;20(6):575–579.
23. Nahata L, Quinn GP, Caltabellotta NM, Tishelman AC. Mental Health Concerns and insurance denials among transgender adolescents. *LGBT Health*. 2017;4.
24. Fertility preservation in patients undergoing gonadotoxic therapy or gonadectomy: a committee opinion. *Fertil Steril*. 2013;100(5):1214–1223.
25. Keene DJ, Sajjad Y, Makin G, Cervellione RM. Sperm banking in the United Kingdom is feasible in patients 13 years old or older with cancer. *J Urol*. 2012;188(2):594–597.
26. Chapple A, Salinas M, Ziebland S, McPherson A, Macfarlane A. Fertility issues: the perceptions and experiences of young men recently diagnosed and treated for cancer. *J Adolesc Health*. 2007;40(1):69–75.
27. Crawshaw MA, Glaser AW, Hale JP, Sloper P. Young males' experiences of sperm banking following a cancer diagnosis—a qualitative study. *Hum Fertil*. 2008;11(4):238–245.
28. Klosky JL, Wang F, Russell KM, et al. Prevalence and predictors of sperm banking in adolescents newly diagnosed with cancer: examination of adolescent, parent, and provider factors influencing fertility preservation outcomes. *J Clin Oncol*. 2017;35.
29. Crawshaw MA, Glaser AW, Pacey AA. The use of pornographic materials by adolescent male cancer patients when banking sperm in the UK: legal and ethical dilemmas. *Hum Fertil*. 2007;10(3):159–163.
30. Adank MC, van Dorp W, Smit M, et al. Electroejaculation as a method of fertility preservation in boys diagnosed with cancer: a single-center experience and review of the literature. *Fertil Steril*. 2014;102(1):199–205.e1.

31. Fullerton G, Hamilton M, Maheshwari A. Should non-mosaic Klinefelter syndrome men be labelled as infertile in 2009? *Hum Reprod.* 2010;25(3):588–597.

32. Moss JL, Choi AW, Fitzgerald Keeter MK, Brannigan RE. Male adolescent fertility preservation. *Fertil Steril.* 2016; 105(2):267–273.

33. Rajfer J. TESA or TESE: which is better for sperm extraction? *Rev Urol.* 2006;8(3):171.

34. Hagenas I, Jorgensen N, Rechnitzer C, et al. Clinical and biochemical correlates of successful semen collection for cryopreservation from 12-18-year-old patients: a single-center study of 86 adolescents. *Hum Reprod.* 2010;25(8): 2031–2038.

35. Wyns C, Curaba M, Vanabelle B, Van Langendonckt A, Donnez J. Options for fertility preservation in prepubertal boys. *Hum Reprod Update.* 2010;16(3):312–328.

36. Keros V, Hultenby K, Borgstrom B, Fridstrom M, Jahnukainen K, Hovattal O. Methods of cryopreservation of testicular tissue with viable spermatogonia in pre-pubertal boys undergoing gonadotoxic cancer treatment. *Hum Reprod.* 2007;22(5):1384–1395.

37. Sato T, Katagiri K, Gohbara A, et al. In vitro production of functional sperm in cultured neonatal mouse testes. *Nature.* 2011;471(7339):504–507.

38. Brinster RL, Zimmermann JW. Spermatogenesis following male germ-cell transplantation. *Proc Natl Acad Sci U S A.* 1994;91(24):11298–11302.

39. Gassei K, Orwig KE. Experimental methods to preserve male fertility and treat male factor infertility. *Fertil Steril.* 2016;105(2):256–266.

40. Yango P, Altman E, Smith JF, Klatsky PC, Tran ND. Optimizing cryopreservation of human spermatogonial stem cells: comparing the effectiveness of testicular tissue and single cell suspension cryopreservation. *Fertil Steril.* 2014;102(5).

41. Practice Committees of American Society for Reproductive Medicine, Society for Assisted Reproductive Technology. Mature oocyte cryopreservation: a guideline. *Fertil Steril.* 2013;99(1):37–43.

42. Oktay K, Bedoschi G. Oocyte cryopreservation for fertility preservation in postpubertal female children at risk for premature ovarian failure due to accelerated follicle loss in Turner syndrome or cancer treatments. *J Pediatr Adolesc Gynecol.* 2014;27(6):342–346.

43. McCracken K, Nahata L. Fertility preservation in children and adolescents: current options and considerations. *Curr Opin Obstet Gynecol.* 2017;29.

44. Hunter MH, Sterrett JJ. Polycystic ovary syndrome: it's not just infertility. *Am Fam Physician.* 2000;62(5):1079–1088.

45. Practice Committee of American Society for Reproductive Medicine. Ovarian tissue cryopreservation: a committee opinion. *Fertil Steril.* 2014;101(5):1237–1243.

46. Hovatta O, Silye R, Krausz T, et al. Cryopreservation of human ovarian tissue using dimethylsulphoxide and propanediol-sucrose as cryoprotectants. *Hum Reprod.* 1996;11(6):1268–1272.

47. Corkum KS, Laronda MM, Rowell EE. A review of re-ported surgical techniques in fertility preservation for prepubertal and adolescent females facing a fertility threatening diagnosis or treatment. *Am J Surg.* 2017; 214(4):695–700.

48. Jensen AK, Macklon KT, Fedder J, Ernst E, Humaidan P, Andersen CY. 86 successful births and 9 ongoing pregnancies worldwide in women transplanted with frozen-thawed ovarian tissue: focus on birth and perinatal outcome in 40 of these children. *J Assist Reprod Genet.* 2017;34(3):325–336.

49. Donnez J, Dolmans MM. Ovarian cortex transplantation: 60 reported live births brings the success and worldwide expansion of the technique towards routine clinical practice. *J Assist Reprod Genet.* 2015;32(8):1167–1170.

50. Donnelly L. Woman gives birth to baby using ovary frozen in her childhood in 'world first'. *Telegraph;* 2016. https://www.telegraph.co.uk/news/2016/12/14/woman-gives-birth-baby-using-ovary-frozen-childhood-inworld/.

51. Bastings L, Beerendonk CC, Westphal JR, et al. Autotrans-plantation of cryopreserved ovarian tissue in cancer survivors and the risk of reintroducing malignancy: a sys-tematic review. *Hum Reprod Update.* 2013;19(5):483–506.

52. Ladanyi C, Mor A, Christianson MS, Dhillon N, Segars JH. Recent advances in the field of ovarian tissue cryopreserva-tion and opportunities for research. *J Assist Reprod Genet.* 2017;34(6):709–722.

53. Shnorhavorian M, Kroon L, Jeffries H, Johnson R. Creating a standardized process to offer the standard of care: contin-uous process improvement methodology is associated with increased rates of sperm cryopreservation among adolescent and young adult males with cancer. *J Pediatr Hematol Oncol.* 2012;34(8):e315–e319.

54. Kelvin JF, Thom B, Benedict C, et al. Cancer and fertility program improves patient satisfaction with information received. *J Clin Oncol.* 2016;34(15):1780–1786.

55. Sheth KR, Sharma V, Helfand BT, et al. Improved fertility preservation care for male patients with cancer after estab-lishment of formalized oncofertility program. *J Urol.* 2012; 187(3):979–986.

56. Chan SW, Cipres D, Katz A, Niemasik EE, Kao CN, Rosen MP. Patient satisfaction is best predicted by low decisional regret among women with cancer seeking fertility preservation counseling (Fpc). *Fertil Steril.* 2014; 102(3):E162–E164.

57. Chong AL, Gupta A, Punnett A, Nathan PC. A cross Canada survey of sperm banking practices in pediatric oncology centers. *Pediatr Blood Cancer.* 2010;55(7):1356–1361.

58. Klosky JL, Anderson LE, Russell KM, et al. Provider influ-ences on sperm banking outcomes among adolescent males newly diagnosed with cancer. *J Adolesc Health.* 2017;60(3):277–283.

59. Stein DM, Victorson DE, Choy JT, et al. Fertility preserva-tion preferences and perspectives among adult male survi-vors of pediatric cancer and their parents. *J Adolesc Young Adult Oncol.* 2014;3(2):75–82.

60. Russell ST, Ryan C, Toomey RB, Diaz RM, Sanchez J. Lesbian, gay, bisexual, and transgender adolescent school victimization: implications for young adult health and adjustment. *J Sch Health*. 2011;81(5):223—230.

61. De Sutter P, Kira K, Verschoor A, Hotimsky A. The desire to have children and the 101 preservation of fertility in transsexual women: a survey. *Int J Transgend*. 2002;6(3).

62. Wierckx K, Van Caenegem E, Pennings G, et al. Reproductive wish in transsexual men. *Hum Reprod*. 2012;27(2):483—487.

63. Tornello SL, Bos H. Parenting intentions among transgender individuals. *LGBT Health*. 2017;4(2):115—120.

64. von Doussa H, Power J, Riggs D. Imagining parenthood: the possibilities and experiences of parenthood among transgender people. *Cult Health Sex*. 2015;17(9):1119—1131.

65. Armuand G, Dhejne C, Olofsson JI, Rodriguez-Wallberg KA. Transgender men's experiences of fertility preservation: a qualitative study. *Hum Reprod*. 2017;32(2):383—390.

66. Maxwell S, Noyes N, Keefe D, Berkeley AS, Goldman KN. Pregnancy outcomes after fertility preservation in transgender men. *Obstet Gynecol*. 2017;129(6):1031—1034.

67. Nahata L, Tishelman AC, Caltabellotta NM, Quinn GP. Low fertility preservation utilization among transgender youth. *J Adolesc Health*. 2017;61.

68. Chen D, Simons L, Johnson EK, Lockart BA, Finlayson C. Fertility preservation for transgender adolescents. *J Adolesc Health*. 2017;61.

69. Strang JF, Jarin J, Call D, et al. Transgender youth fertility attitudes questionnaire: measure development in nonautistic and autistic transgender youth and their parents. *J Adolesc Health*. 2017;62.

70. Olson KR, Durwood L, DeMeules M, McLaughlin KA. Mental health of transgender children who are supported in their identities. *Pediatrics*. 2016;137(3):e20153223.

71. Tishelman AC, Kaufman R, Edwards-Leeper L, Mandel FH, Shumer DE, Spack NP. Serving transgender youth: challenges, dilemmas and clinical examples. *Prof Psychol Res Pr*. 2015;46(1):37—45.

72. Reisner SL, Vetters R, Leclerc M, et al. Mental health of transgender youth in care at an adolescent urban community health center: a matched retrospective cohort study. *J Adolesc Health*. 2015;56(3):274—279.

73. Shumer DE, Reisner SL, Edwards-Leeper L, Tishelman A. Evaluation of asperger syndrome in youth presenting to a gender dysphoria clinic. *LGBT Health*. 2016;3(5):387—390.

74. Strang JF, Meagher H, Kenworthy L, et al. Initial clinical guidelines for co-occurring autism spectrum disorder and gender dysphoria or incongruence in adolescents. *J Clin Child Adolesc Psychol*. 2016;47:1—11.

75. Shumer DE, Tishelman AC. The role of assent in the treatment of transgender adolescents. *Int J Transgend*. 2015;16(2):97—102.

76. Bensing JM, Deveugele M, Moretti F, et al. How to make the medical consultation more successful from a patient's perspective? Tips for doctors and patients from lay people in the United Kingdom, Italy, Belgium and The Netherlands. *Patient Educ Couns*. 2011;84(3):287—293.

77. McDougall RJ, Gillam L, Delany C, Jayasinghe Y. Ethics of fertility preservation for prepubertal children: should clinicians offer procedures where efficacy is largely unproven? *J Med Ethics*. 2017;44.

78. Loren AW, Mangu PB, Beck LN, et al. Fertility preservation for patients with cancer: American Society of Clinical Oncology clinical practice guideline update. *J Clin Oncol*. 2013;31(19):2500—2510.

79. Katz AL, Webb SA, Committee On Bioethics. Informed consent in decision-making in pediatric practice. *Pediatrics*. 2016;138(2).

80. Quinn GP, Murphy D, Knapp C, et al. Who decides? Decision making and fertility preservation in teens with cancer: a review of the literature. *J Adolesc Health*. 2011;49(4):337—346.

81. Grossman AH, D'Augelli AR, Howell TJ, Hubbard S. Parent' reactions to transgender youth' gender nonconforming expression and identity. *J Gay Lesbian Soc Serv*. 2005;18(1).

82. Nahata L, Campo-Engelstein L, Tishelman AC, Quinn GP, Lantos J. Ethics rounds: fertility preservation for a transgender teen. Pediatrics. In Press.

83. Mersereau JE, Goodman LR, Deal AM, Gorman JR, Whitcomb BW, Su HI. To preserve or not to preserve: how difficult is the decision about fertility preservation? *Cancer*. 2013;119(22):4044—4050.

84. Cardozo ER, Huber WJ, Stuckey AR, Alvero RJ. Mandating coverage for fertility preservation—a step in the right direction. *New Engl J Med*. 2017;377(17):1607—1609.

85. Levine J, Canada A, Stern CJ. Fertility preservation in adolescents and young adults with cancer. *J Clin Oncol*. 2010;28(32):4831—4841.

CHAPTER 10

Duration of Pubertal Suppression and Initiation of Gender-Affirming Hormone Treatment in Youth

HADRIAN MYLES KINNEAR, BA • DANIEL EVAN SHUMER, MD, MPH

Gender identity describes a person's deeply held feelings of being a boy or girl, man or woman, or another nonbinary understanding of their gender.[1] The adolescent with gender dysphoria has a gender identity incongruent with their sex assigned at birth causing distress.[2] Current management of children and adolescents with gender dysphoria has its roots in the so-called "Dutch Protocol", whereby puberty was suppressed at pubertal (Tanner) stage 2, followed by treatment with gender-affirming hormones later in adolescence.[3] In this way, the transgender adolescent was treated sequentially with medications which had been previously used for both precocious puberty and for delayed puberty.[4,5]

The "Dutch Protocol" was subsequently used as a basis for recommendations outlined by professional organizations such as the World Professional Association for Transgender Health (WPATH) and the Endocrine Society. The WPATH Standards of Care (SOC) for the Health of Transsexual, Transgender, and Gender-Nonconforming People (version 7, 2012)[6] and the Endocrine Society Clinical Practice Guideline for Endocrine Treatment of Gender-Dysphoric/Gender-Incongruent Persons (2017)[7] outline treatment recommendations pertaining to the use of these medical interventions. However, since the "Dutch Protocol" was first described, there have been dramatic shifts in how transgender and gender-nonconforming youth are accessing care, and how individuals are conceptualizing gender. For example, patients who fit the treatment paradigm initially described by the Dutch had gender dysphoria presenting prior to the start of puberty. In practice, the majority of adolescents present to clinic later than pubertal stage 2.[8] In addition, individuals are increasingly expanding beyond the male/female, boy/girl, man/woman binary ideas of sex and

gender.[9] In parallel, estimates of the prevalence of transgender identities are rapidly changing. Previous estimates using data from the 1970s calculated the prevalence of transgender identities at 1:30,000 for natal males, and 1:100,000 for natal females;[10] however, an adult sample from Massachusetts placed the combined estimate at 0.5% in 2012.[11] This 2012 finding has been further supported by two groups using data from the 2014 US Centers for Disease Control and Prevention Behavioral Risk Factor Surveillance System to place the estimates at 0.53%[12] and 0.6%[13] of the US population (1.4 million US adults). Furthermore, at our children's hospital-based gender clinic, consultations with transgender boys now outpace consultations with transgender girls at a rate of 2:1, a ratio anecdotally similar to peer institutions. Finally, pubertal suppression medications as well as most other treatment used in the "Dutch Protocol" were covered by their national insurance program, whereas this very expensive medication may or may not be covered by current health insurance depending on the area of practice.[14] In addition, an implicit assumption was made that transgender adults would (1) desire and (2) be able to afford gonadectomy, whereas in clinical practice neither one of these assumptions may be true.

As the field of transgender medicine works to keep pace with epidemiologic shifts and social changes, clinicians are left with clinical questions, which may not be adequately outlined by current guidelines and SOC. Central to these clinical questions remain the following:

1. When should a patient begin pubertal suppression treatment?
2. When should a patient begin gender-affirming hormones?
3. When should a patient discontinue use of pubertal suppression treatment?

The goal of this chapter is to outline and contextualize current treatments and protocols, explore primary research around these topics, and provide a series of case examples for multiple clinical situations.

PUBERTAL SUPPRESSION AND GENDER-AFFIRMING HORMONE THERAPIES

The hypothalamus produces spikes of gonadotropin-releasing hormone (GnRH), which stimulates the pituitary to produce pulsatile luteinizing hormone (LH) and follicle-stimulating hormone (FSH), in turn stimulating the gonads. Specifically, LH stimulates the Leydig cells in the testes to produce testosterone and the thecal cells in the ovary to produce androgens which are converted to estradiol in granulosa cells.[15] The model for pubertal suppression treatment uses GnRH agonists, commonly leuprolide acetate and histrelin acetate, which are generally used for precocious puberty.[16] GnRH agonists work by providing a basal level of GnRH, which, somewhat counterintuitively, inhibits the pituitary secretion of LH and FSH. In turn, the production of the sex steroids in the gonads is suppressed.[17]

Following pubertal suppression with GnRH agonists, gender-affirming hormone therapy with sex steroids is used for pubertal induction. Transmasculine individuals are typically prescribed testosterone either as a parenteral testosterone ester or transdermal testosterone gel or patch. Transfeminine individuals are typically prescribed estrogen (oral, transdermal, or parenteral) in addition to an antiandrogen or a GnRH agonist.[7] Gender-affirming hormones are used for pubertal induction and then continued indefinitely into adulthood.

Inhibition of sex hormone production by administration of GnRH agonists can serve three proximal goals in hormonal management of transgender persons. First, the development of isosexual secondary sex characteristics can be inhibited. Second, reduction in isosexual sex hormones may make use of cross-sex hormones more effective at promoting a hormonal transition, or may make the required dosage of cross-sex hormones for effective transition lower and perhaps safer. In our practice, this "block and replace" strategy is used primarily in transgender women, who may have more successful and safe feminization on a GnRH agonist plus low-dose estrogen compared to higher dose estrogen without a GnRH agonist. Third, the effects of ongoing production of isosexual sex hormones in a transgender person, which may be causing dysphoric symptoms in a pubertal or postpubertal person, could be reduced. Examples of this include suppression of testosterone in a transgender woman who is experiencing dysphoric erections, or the suppression of estrogen in a transgender man who is experiencing dysphoric menses.

In practice, the use of GnRH agonists is often complicated by cost and insurance coverage. Therefore, there may be more notable benefits for use of GnRH agonists in some situations when compared to others, and this may have logistical impacts on practice. For example, a transgender boy at the start of puberty (early breast budding) would have a significant benefit from a GnRH agonist with no suitable alternative if the goal is to prevent development of breasts. Alternatively, a transgender boy at pubertal stage 5 (full breast development) could theoretically use a GnRH agonist to suppress menses while considering starting testosterone. However, this patient could alternatively trial simpler approaches to suppress menses, such as depo-medroxyprogesterone, or a daily oral progestin (Fig. 10.1).

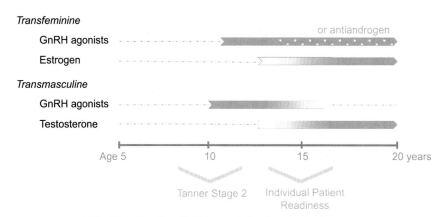

FIG. 10.1 Timeline. *GnRH*, gonadotropin-releasing hormone.

RELEVANT TIME POINTS IN CLINICAL GUIDELINES AND PROTOCOLS

Clinicians and patients considering pubertal suppression need to decide when to (1) start GnRH agonist treatments, (2) start gender-affirming sex steroid treatment, (3) stop GnRH agonist treatments, and (4) when to consider alternative approaches if GnRH agonist treatments are not available to an individual patient. Each of these questions requires consideration of the goals of therapy for the individual patient.

We will examine how current clinical guidelines and protocols address these specific time points. We will compare the "Dutch Protocol", the WPATH SOC (version 7), the University of California San Francisco's (UCSF) primary care guidelines, and the 2017 Endocrine Society Clinical Practice Guidelines.

The "Dutch Protocol"

The seminal work around pubertal suppression for transgender youth occurred in the Netherlands. The timeline set forth by the Amsterdam Gender Clinic in 2006 was as follows: eligible adolescents may begin GnRH agonists at Tanner stage 2 or 3 *and* older than 12 years.[3] In the Netherlands, the age of 12 years was chosen as an age when adolescents may make medical decisions together with their caretakers.[18] The assumption was made that the onset of puberty helps to clarify whether gender dysphoria will persist. Additionally, they noted that this protocol could be applied to adolescents in later phases of pubertal development to halt future progression of puberty. At the age of 16 years, sex steroids were initiated, followed by the option for genital surgery and gonad removal at the age of 18 years. Sixteen years of age was established for beginning sex steroid hormone therapy, as 16-year-olds are considered legal adults for medical decision-making in the Netherlands. Gender-affirming pubertal development was initiated by the use of increasing sex steroid dosage every 6 months until the adult dose was reached. GnRH agonist treatment was continued at least until maintenance level of sex steroids was reached with a preference to continue until gonadectomy. Additionally, in 2006 in the Netherlands, changing the birth certificate (the source for other personal documents) was only possible after the patient had their gonads removed.[3] However, as of 2014, it is now possible to change official documents in the Netherlands without gonadectomy. In qualitative analyses of transgender youth in the Netherlands, statements such as the following were documented: "I don't care about hysterectomy because changing gender on official documents is nowadays possible without this surgical procedure"

(p. 1701),[19] highlighting the intersection between the medical and legal spheres.

In review of the "Dutch Protocol," some important considerations are worth addressing. First, the Dutch authors did make note that provision of hormonal treatment to adolescents is a controversial topic. Despite the controversy, Cohen-Kettenis et al., in 2008, made the case that nonintervention is not a neutral decision for a clinician.[20] Second, the societal and legal context in the Netherlands helped to frame how different ages were selected for making treatment decisions. As much of the published literature around pubertal suppression came from the Netherlands, other clinicians began to benchmark their timing toward similar ages: Tanner stage 2 or 3 *and* 12 years of age for starting GnRH agonists, gender-affirming hormones not until at age of 16 years, and continuation of GnRH agonist treatment with removal of the gonads not before the age of 18 years. That said, the use of age cutoffs for what are essentially decisions predicated on patient and family readiness may or may not make sense in modern contexts. Finally, it is worth restating that nearly all gender-affirming treatment was covered by insurance in the Netherlands resulting in limited consideration to costs for these interventions.[21]

World Professional Association for Transgender Health

The WPATH SOC is based on professional consensus using the best data available to provide flexible guidelines for clinicians. Originally published in 1979, the current version (version 7) was published in 2012. The SOC separates treatments for adolescents into fully reversible (pubertal suppression), partially reversible (sex steroids), and irreversible (surgical) interventions. Fully reversible interventions intend to delay or suppress puberty and often include GnRH agonists. Other reversible medications include progestins (medroxyprogesterone) and spironolactone (to decrease androgen effects). WPATH comments on two relevant time points: (1) starting puberty suppression and (2) starting sex steroid therapy. Puberty-suppressing hormone eligibility may begin as soon as adolescents have the onset of puberty to Tanner stage 2, which they note may occur as early as 9 years of age, although it is stated that the evaluation of this approach has only been studied for adolescents who were at least 12 years old. The goals of suppression include giving more time for the adolescent to explore gender while preventing difficult-to-reverse development of secondary sex characteristics. For timing of gender-affirming hormones, the WPATH SOC offers more general guidance, noting that the age of consent may be relevant, as well as hormone regimens adapted to account for adolescent development. Additionally, little is offered around the appropriate time to stop treatment with GnRH agonist medication. GnRH agonists are also mentioned for adult endogenous hormone suppression, on a list of possible antiandrogens for use in transgender women and in the context of masculinizing hormone therapy for transgender men to assist with menstrual cessation if needed.[6]

University of California San Francisco Primary Care Guidelines

Johanna Olson-Kennedy, Stephen Rosenthal, Jennifer Hastings, and Linda Wesp authored the section of the UCSF Guidelines for Primary and Gender-Affirming Care of Transgender and Gender Nonbinary People entitled "Health considerations for gender nonconforming children and transgender adolescents" (p. 186).[22] In understanding the medical care for transgender youth, they separate youth into two cohorts— early pubertal youth (Tanner stages 2–3) and late pubertal youth (Tanner stages 4–5). They note that GnRH agonists are ideally initiated at the earliest stages of puberty (Tanner 2–3) to avoid development of undesired secondary sexual characteristics and discuss that there is limited study on administration of GnRH agonists at younger than 12 years of age. The UCSF Primary Care Guidelines note that the onset of puberty may occur much sooner than 12 years of age,[22] drawing on the work of Biro et al. demonstrating that at the age of 7 years, 10% of white, 23% of black non-Hispanic, and 15% of Hispanic girls had obtained breast stage ≥Tanner stage 2.[23]

With respect to the initiation of gender-affirming hormones, the UCSF Guidelines discuss consideration of hormone initiation prior to the age of 16 years related to several factors. These include the length of time on a GnRH agonist as potentially relevant to bone density, the upheaval that may come from experiencing puberty in late high school or early college, and data suggesting that youth who reach adolescence and experience gender dysphoria are likely to persist.[22] This persistence is supported by findings that pubertal suppression did not ameliorate gender dysphoria for the first 70 eligible candidates treated at the Amsterdam gender identity clinic of the VU University Medical Center.[24]

The discontinuation of GnRH agonists is also discussed in regard to the "Dutch Protocol," which historically has aligned this to gonadectomy. Genital surgeries and gonadectomy may be more complicated to obtain and afford in the United States and other countries, and also may not be desirable for many transgender individuals. These guidelines discuss potential continuation of a GnRH agonist concurrently with gender-affirming hormones into late adolescence or early adulthood, particularly to reduce required doses of estradiol in transgender girls. Finally, the UCSF Guidelines discusses strategies for the management of hormone therapy, particularly for late pubertal use, with or without the use of GnRH agonists.[22]

Endocrine Society Clinical Practice Guidelines

The Endocrine Society offers updated clinical practice guidelines published in September 2017. These guidelines recommend treating gender-dysphoric/gender-incongruent adolescents with GnRH agonists when they have reached Tanner stage 2. Tanner stage 2 is defined as "breast and papilla elevated as small mound; areolar diameter increased"; and "slight enlargement of penis, enlarged scrotum, pink, texture altered, testes 4–6 mL" (p. 13).[7]

Regarding initiation of gender-affirming hormones, the clinical guidelines dictate that clinicians may begin sex steroids after a multidisciplinary team confirms persistent gender dysphoria/gender incongruence and the patient has sufficient mental capacity for informed consent. It is noted that there may be "compelling reasons" (p. 2) for beginning treatment with sex steroids before the age of 16 years, although there has been limited literature published on treating patients prior to 13.5/14 years of age.[7]

These guidelines also note that rigorous study and evaluation is needed to determine the effects of prolonged pubertal delay on bones, gonads, and brain development. Additionally, they highlight that GnRH agonists are the preferred treatment option (there are also GnRH antagonists without sufficient data around their safety and efficacy in adolescents). The Endocrine Society guidelines list the time to stop GnRH agonist treatment as gonadectomy, although it is acknowledged that this may not be a procedure chosen by the patient. The alternative time points for stopping GnRH agonist treatment include once the adult dose of testosterone has been reached in transgender men. However, it is noted that combined testosterone and GnRH agonists could potentially allow for lower doses of testosterone. For discontinuing GnRH agonist treatment in transgender women, it is noted that some adjunctive therapy is needed in addition to physiologic doses of estrogen and that other antiandrogens may be used, such as spironolactone and cyproterone acetate in addition to

Guidelines	Start GnRH agonists	Start Sex Steroids	Stop GnRH agonists
Dutch Protocol (2006)[3]	Tanner stage 2 or 3 and older than 12 years	Age of 16 years	Gonadectomy (eligible at 18 years of age)
WPATH SOC (2012)[6]	Tanner stage 2	Relevant to age of consent and adolescent development	Unclear, may be used in adults
UCSF Primary Care Guidelines (2016)[22]	Tanner stage 2	Consider prior to 16 years of age relevant to bone density & upheaval of late puberty	Can continue into adulthood, particularly for trans-feminine individuals
Endocrine Society Clinical Practice Guidelines (2017)[7]	Tanner stage 2	May treat before the age of 16 years, limited literature prior to 13.5/14 years	At gonadectomy *or* Transmasculine: adult dose of testosterone reached; Transfeminine: use with estrogen or replace with other antiandrogen

FIG. 10.2 Guidance summary diagram.

GnRH agonists.[7] It should be noted that cyproterone acetate is not available for use in the United States (Fig. 10.2).

UNRESOLVED QUESTIONS

The four guidelines discussed above (Dutch Protocol, WPATH, UCSF, and Endocrine Society) are clear on the use of GnRH agonist medications beginning in early puberty. This treatment forestalls the onset of secondary sex characteristics, avoiding the accompanying dysphoria of this development in the transgender child. In addition, the older transgender adolescent or adult who never developed secondary sex characteristics of their sex assigned at birth may have a more straightforward time presenting themselves as their affirmed gender. Finally, the treatment allows for protected time to explore gender and to make a balanced decision on the use of gender-affirming hormones in later adolescence. However, the published guidelines offer less nuance and guidance around topics commonly encountered when treating transgender youth. For example, if GnRH agonists are started in early puberty, when should they be discontinued, especially if gonadectomy is not practical or desired? What about the large percentage of adolescents seeking medical care well after the onset of puberty—are GnRH agonists helpful for these patients? If so, should GnRH agonists be considered for adult transgender patients presenting for care?

While peer-reviewed studies attempting to tackle these questions are sparse, we've attempted to guide the reader through the various situations when GnRH agonists could be considered, and when the use of GnRH agonists may or may not be helpful. In writing this section, we have relied on personal clinical experience, input from other experts in the field, published clinical guidance, and the limited available data on medical treatment and outcomes for transgender individuals.

CASE EXAMPLES
Case 1: the 9-Year-Old Prepubertal Boy or Girl at Pubertal Stage 1

Families of transgender or gender nonconforming youth may present to primary care providers or multidisciplinary gender clinics looking for guidance on topics related to gender. For example, a 9-year-old and their parents may present to their primary care provider to discuss the right timing to make a social transition. The family may request referral to a therapist with experience in gender to help sort through topics of gender exploration, or to navigate challenges related to making a social transition. Often, we see prepubertal children referred to our multidisciplinary gender clinic. These children will undergo a comprehensive gender and psychosocial assessment by one of our clinic's mental health professionals. The clinician will provide gender-related education and support to the family, and also to the child at an age-appropriate level. There may be a recommendation to connect with a therapist in the patient's community with experience in gender, or referral to a psychiatrist if the child has comorbid psychopathology such as anxiety or depression that may require a medical intervention. The family may also wish to meet with one of the clinic's physicians for discussion of hormonal interventions for gender dysphoria. Additionally, the family may not know whether the child is perhaps in early puberty, and a careful pubertal staging exam is required.

The current guidance from WPATH and the Endocrine Society does not support treatment of prepubertal youth with GnRH agonists for purposes of pubertal suppression. Treatment before pubertal stage 2 is not necessary, as pubertal hormone production does not yet occur prior to this stage. Furthermore, it is thought that early puberty can have some diagnostic value—if gender dysphoria persists or intensifies in early puberty, it is more likely to persist as adolescence continues; if it dissipates, then treatment may not be necessary. In a Dutch study aimed toward understanding persistence of gender dysphoria, older children were found to be more likely to persist.[25] Furthermore, some of the changes in early puberty up to Tanner stage 2 show regression with GnRH agonists, including reductions in testicular volume and varying degrees of breast development regression.[26]

In medical visits with prepubertal youth, it is our practice to discuss topics of gender including validating the child's gender experience, assessing mental health needs, and providing information at an age-appropriate level about puberty and the option of intervention with pubertal suppression in the future. A pubertal staging exam can be performed to confirm that the child remains at pubertal stage 1. Frequency of visits can vary depending on the age of the child. A very young child may not need to see a hormone provider for years and can continue to follow with their supportive primary care provider. Peripubertal children could be followed at closer intervals for pubertal staging exams, or this could be accomplished using a team approach with the primary care provider. Parents and children can also be given guidance on contacting their health professional if they note early breast development or testicular enlargement, the hallmarks of pubertal stage 2, between visits, with instruction to contact the office should these findings develop. Parents

anxious to avoid even the very start of puberty may request GnRH agonist treatment for their child prior to the start of puberty; however, this is not the recommended treatment by current guidelines, and it is not our practice to intervene in this manner.

Case 2: the 11-Year-Old Transgender Boy at Pubertal Stage 2

Breast budding is the hallmark of pubertal stage 2 in natal females. The average age of breast budding (pubertal stage 2) varies throughout the population and ranges from 8.9 to 11.2 years across studies.[27] The current definition of precocious puberty in natal females is the onset of central puberty prior to 8 years of age[28]; the definition of delayed puberty is the lack of central puberty at the age of 13 years.[29] The transgender boy who is currently at pubertal stage 2 and meets criteria for gender dysphoria is eligible to receive pubertal suppression using a GnRH agonist.[6,7]

There are several rationales for treatment. Continued development of secondary sexual characteristics can exacerbate gender dysphoria. Additionally, development of secondary sex characteristics that are permanent may require surgical treatment in the future. Specifically, treatment with GnRH agonists at pubertal stage 2, followed by future treatment with testosterone, can obviate the potential need for masculinizing chest surgery. Furthermore, because GnRH agonist therapy is considered a "reversible" intervention (i.e., puberty would commence if the medication is discontinued), the adolescent can continue to explore their gender identity prior to making a commitment to the "partially irreversible" intervention of testosterone therapy.

When starting GnRH agonist therapy in a transgender boy at pubertal stage 2, multiple important considerations should be explored. First, the child and family should be counseled that the treatment will affect the normal timing of the pubertal growth spurt. Children treated with GnRH agonists continue to grow at a prepubertal speed. It would be expected that growth acceleration would commence once the child is withdrawn from GnRH agonist therapy, or once testosterone treatment is initiated. Preliminary study has shown slowed height velocity gain during pubertal suppression, with growth spurts shown after administration of testosterone but not estrogen.[3]

Second, bone metabolism is affected by pubertal suppression. Pubertal hormones are important modulators of the relative increase in bone strength that occurs in adolescence. Bone density accrual will continue in a prepubertal fashion while on treatment; however, the adolescent acceleration in bone density will be postponed until withdrawal from GnRH agonist medication or treatment with testosterone. Experiences of the first 21 patients treated with the Dutch Protocol demonstrated no significant changes (although reduced calculated z-score) in bone mineral density during pubertal suppression for the lumbar spine, femoral neck, and total body. Significant increases in bone density were also shown following sex steroid treatment.[3] Another longitudinal study demonstrated reduction in lumbar spine absolute bone mineral density z-scores for 34 adolescents (using natal sex reference values) when compared prior to the start of GnRH agonists and then for follow-up at the age of 22 years (after treatment with GnRH agonists, sex steroids, and gonadectomy). These findings were interpreted to be related to delayed or reduced peak bone mass potential.[30]

Third, menarche will not occur while on treatment with a GnRH agonist. This is likely reassuring to transgender boys. However, this eliminates the potential for oocyte harvesting in interested patients by controlled ovarian stimulation. Fertility preservation in a prepubertal female is not a standardly available procedure, as ovarian tissue cryopreservation is currently considered experimental, although it may be moving toward broader clinical implementation.[31] Therefore, while treatment with GnRH agonist does not, itself, cause infertility, the patient may be progressing down a road toward possible infertility by embarking on GnRH agonist therapy prior to menarche with the intention of future sex steroid treatment. Fertility for transgender men on sex steroid treatment (testosterone) has not been well studied. Current guidelines assume loss of fertility with testosterone treatment and encourage prior oocyte or embryo cryopreservation.[7] Despite assumed fertility loss, there are accounts in the literature where some transgender men have paused testosterone and carried pregnancies, while others have unintentionally become pregnant while taking testosterone therapy.[32]

Finally, there are several other health considerations for transgender adolescents considering GnRH agonist therapy. There have been several reported cases in the literature of GnRH agonist-induced arterial hypertension in transgender boys.[33] Additionally, fat percentage increased and lean body mass percentage decreased during the first year of treatment with GnRH agonists for both transgender boys and transgender girls.[26] Therefore, in review of these multiple important considerations, careful discussion of the risks and benefits of GnRH agonist therapy is necessary before proceeding.

The transgender boy who starts on GnRH agonists at pubertal stage 2 becomes eligible for testosterone treatment later in adolescence provided that their gender identity as a boy persists over time. Timing of testosterone therapy is debated. Historically, 16 years of age had been used, correlating to the Dutch age of consent. However, the psychological impact of delaying puberty to the age of 16 years can be challenging for transgender boys who are watching their peers complete puberty by this age. Contemporary practice in the United States is trending toward clinicians being primarily focused on patient readiness, maturity, and the ability to understand risks and benefits of testosterone treatment. The 2017 version of the Endocrine Society Clinical Practice Guideline recognizes that there may be reasons to begin sex hormone treatment before the age of 16 years, with the acknowledgement that there are limited published studies prior to the age of 13.5−14 years.[7]

A transgender adolescent boy on testosterone may no longer require GnRH agonist medication. The suppressive effect of testosterone on the adolescent's hypothalamic−pituitary−ovarian axis may obviate the need for concurrent treatment with a GnRH agonist and testosterone. It is therefore our practice to discontinue GnRH agonist therapy once testosterone dosing is increased to the adult dose. The estradiol level and clinical exam can guide whether discontinuation of a GnRH agonist after initiation of testosterone level is effective. Estradiol levels in the female range or clinical progression of breast development may necessitate an increase in the testosterone dose or resumption of GnRH agonist therapy. If GnRH agonist therapy is needed concurrently with testosterone treatment, it could be discontinued if the patient elects for hysterectomy/oophorectomy as an adult.

In some instances, a natal female on GnRH agonist therapy may express a desire to continue GnRH agonist therapy indefinitely, rather than discontinue it and proceed through female puberty or start testosterone. This desire may be founded on a rejection of a binary gender identity or identification as agender. While understandable, the importance of pubertal hormones for physical health and bone health necessitate that adolescents do get exposure to puberty. The indefinite withholding of puberty is not recommended.

Case 3: the 11-Year-Old Transgender Girl at Pubertal Stage 2

Testicular enlargement is the hallmark of pubertal stage 2 in natal males. Testicular enlargement occurs due to stimulation of the testes by gonadotropins and is accompanied by testosterone production. This pubertal stage is often less obvious to patients and parents than breast budding in natal females. For this reason, pubertal staging exams by a physician can be helpful in the identification of the start of male puberty in transgender girls. The average age of testicular enlargement >3 mL was reported to be 11.6 years, with a range of 9.6–13.7 years in a recent Danish study.[34] Similarly, the average age for genital Tanner stage 2 was 10.1, 9.1, and 10.0 years in non-Hispanic white, African-American, and Hispanic youth, respectively, as found by an office-based study from the American Academy of Pediatrics.[35] Precocious puberty in natal males is defined as the onset prior to the age of 9 years, and delayed puberty is defined as no pubertal development by the age of 14 years.[28,29]

Transgender girls at pubertal stage 2 are eligible for treatment with a GnRH agonist. Rationales for treatment are similar to the rationales for transgender boys. Continued development of male secondary sexual characteristics may exacerbate gender dysphoria. Many of these changes, such as the deepening of the voice and development of a prominent Adam's apple, growth of facial and body hair, and masculinization of the face, would be permanent. The intervention with a GnRH agonist is "reversible" and allows time for further gender identity exploration prior to committing to feminizing medications.

Initiation of treatment with a GnRH agonist in a transgender girl at pubertal stage 2 requires discussion about several other considerations. The adolescent will continue to grow, but at a prepubertal speed, while on GnRH agonist therapy. If estrogen is initiated later in adolescence, a growth spurt and subsequent growth arrest will occur, likely resulting in a shorter final adult height than if no intervention was pursued. Similarly to transgender boys, bone density accrual will continue in a prepubertal fashion while on treatment; however, the adolescent acceleration in bone density will be postponed until withdrawal from GnRH agonist medication or treatment with estrogen. Spermatogenesis will not occur if puberty is suppressed.[36] Therefore, a child treated with GnRH agonist medication followed by estrogen would not have the opportunity to preserve sperm using the standard methods.

The transgender girl who starts on GnRH agonist therapy at pubertal stage 2 would become eligible for estrogen treatment in later adolescence if her gender identity as a girl persists. As discussed in Case 2, the age of initiation of estrogen treatment was historically set at 16 years, but there has been a shift toward treatment at younger ages based on individual patient readiness.

After initiation of estrogen, the transgender girl may benefit from continued pubertal suppression using a GnRH agonist—a departure from the guidance for transgender boys. Concurrent treatment with a GnRH agonist plus estradiol, the so-called "block and replace" strategy, allows for smaller doses of estrogen to achieve normal female puberty. In our experience, the dose of estradiol required for normal female puberty in a patient on concurrent GnRH agonist treatment is similar to the dosing used in cisgender girls with ovarian insufficiency—oral 17-β estradiol, 2 mg orally daily, or transdermal estradiol patches 0.1 mg/24 h. This is in contrast to much higher doses often required in transgender girls not on GnRH agonist treatment—oral 17-β estradiol 6–8 mg orally daily, or transdermal estradiol patches up to 0.4 mg/24 h.[22] When treating a transgender adolescent or young adult with estrogen, the Endocrine Society suggests goals of therapy as maintaining a serum estradiol level between 100 and 200 pg/mL, and a serum testosterone level less than 50 ng/dL.[7] It is clear that achieving these goals is easier when using the "block and replace" strategy. That said, in practice, as previously stated, GnRH agonist medications are expensive and often insurance coverage is difficult to obtain. For this reason, we often advocate strongly for coverage for the transgender girl at pubertal stage 2 *at least* until estrogen treatment commences, and then continue treatment with a GnRH agonist if possible, but with less urgency.

In the patient with initiation of GnRH agonist treatment at pubertal stage 2, followed by continued concurrent treatment with GnRH agonist and estrogen treatment in later adolescence, the GnRH agonist treatment could be discontinued at the time of gonadectomy, if surgery is desired in young adulthood. There is some concern that technical aspects of vaginoplasty are made more difficult when the surgery is performed on a young adult who has never gone through male puberty—the phallic size is smaller in these patients, and there is less tissue available for certain surgical methods used to create the neovagina.[20]

As outlined in Case 2, there may be instances where a natal male on GnRH agonist therapy may express a desire to continue GnRH agonist therapy indefinitely, without proceeding through male puberty or starting estrogen. Again, the importance of pubertal hormones for physical health and bone health necessitate that adolescents do get exposure to puberty, and indefinite withholding of puberty is not recommended.

Case 4: the 15-Year-Old Transgender Boy at Pubertal Stage 4

Many transgender adolescents do not present for care at the time of onset of puberty. In our clinic, for example, approximately two-thirds of patients are presenting for care at pubertal stage 4 or 5. A transgender boy presenting at pubertal stage 4 requires different medical considerations than a transgender boy presenting at pubertal stage 2. The most obvious physical difference between stage 4 and 2 is breast development. The transgender boy at pubertal stage 4 has breasts nearing adult size and contour. The adolescent is likely menarchal, and if not, will be having menarche soon.

In considering treatment options for the transgender boy at pubertal stage 4, one must first consider goals of treatment. Goals may include (1) to start a masculinizing puberty, (2) to stop menses or prevent menses from starting, and (3) to limit further breast development.

The patient may or may not be ready to start treatment testosterone. If the adolescent meets readiness criteria for initiation of testosterone, we recommend starting testosterone and not initiating treatment with a GnRH agonist (see Case 2). If the adolescent is not ready to start testosterone treatment, GnRH agonist medication would be helpful in suppressing menses and limiting further breast development. That said, breast development already present would not resolve, and masculinizing chest surgery would likely still be required in the future for chest-based dysphoria. In addition, there are other hormonal methods that could be employed to suppress menses besides GnRH agonist treatment. In this situation, given the high cost of GnRH agonist medication for marginal utility, we employ progesterone for purposes of menstrual suppression in the late-pubertal transgender boy not ready for testosterone treatment. Norethindrone or other progestin-only oral pills, or depo-medroxyprogesterone acetate 150 mg intramuscularly every 3 months can be used in this patient population with the primary goal of suppression of dysphoric menses.[37] If testosterone treatment is subsequently initiated, progesterone treatment can be discontinued.

Case 5: the 15-Year-Old Transgender Girl at Pubertal Stage 4

Likewise, a transgender girl presenting at pubertal stage 4 requires different medical considerations than a transgender girl presenting at pubertal stage 2. This patient will have had almost complete masculinization of the external genitalia and deepening of the voice. However, there are several important processes that occur in late male puberty that are of significant consequence to the transgender girl. First, fullness of facial hair and body hair are late-developing processes in male puberty.

Second, full masculinization of the face is another late-developing process, such that natal males with almost complete pubertal genital development, or even natal males at genital stage 5, often have a young appearing face, which will continue to masculinize into late adolescence and early adulthood. Therefore, we are more aggressive in our attempt to treat transgender girls in later puberty with GnRH agonist medications. As outlined in Case 3, we would consider treatment with GnRH agonist regardless of whether estrogen was being initiated concurrently for these patients and consider continuing this treatment until gonadectomy if desired in young adulthood, and dependent on their ability to obtain coverage for the medication.

Spironolactone, a weak androgen receptor antagonist, can also be used in this patient population if GnRH agonists are not used. The medication, prescribed at dosing ranging from 100 to 300 mg/day orally,[7] blunts the effect of androgens and can be helpful at slowing development of unwanted facial and body hair, or other masculinizing effects of male puberty. Other medications that suppress androgen action, including cyproterone acetate, flutamide, nilutamide, and bicalutamide, have been reported for use in transgender women as well.[38]

Case 6: the 17-Year-Old Transgender Boy at Pubertal Stage 5, or the Adult Transgender Man

Treatment considerations for the postpubertal transgender boy are similar to considerations for the transgender boy presenting at pubertal stage 4. Monotherapy with testosterone could be considered based on patient readiness. Progesterones could be considered for menstrual suppression for patients with dysphoric menses not ready for testosterone treatment.

Case 7: the 17-Year-Old Transgender Girl at Pubertal Stage 5, or the Adult Transgender Woman

Treatment considerations for the postpubertal transgender girl are similar to considerations for the transgender girl presenting at pubertal stage 4. Estrogen can be started based on patient readiness. Adjunctive treatment with a GnRH agonist can be helpful, if available, using the "block and replace" strategy described in Case 3. If GnRH agonists are not used, and especially if monotherapy with estrogen is not achieving adequate clinical results and/or ideal blood levels of estrogen and testosterone, adjunctive therapy with antiandrogens can also be considered (i.e., spironolactone, cyproterone acetate, bicalutamide. When GnRH agonists are used in conjunction with estrogen, this intervention could be discontinued at the time of gonadectomy, if desired.

Case 8: The Gender Nonconforming Child in Early Puberty

Gender nonconforming children are increasingly presenting to gender clinics to discuss treatment with GnRH agonist medications. For example, a natal male or a natal female may present to the clinic at the age of 13 years after parental discussion around their identification as genderqueer. Some parents may research interventions and request GnRH agonist medications while their child works through their gender identity. In our experience, the current generation of youth is expanding the boundaries of sexuality and gender, and often times rejecting binary ideas of gender, sex, and sexuality. This requires careful consideration by clinicians as to when medical intervention is appropriate.

We define gender identity as a deeply held internal sense of oneself as a boy or girl, man or woman, another gender (e.g., genderqueer, nonbinary), or no gender at all (e.g., agender). Gender expression is the way one manifests one's gender by the way that one acts, dresses, and presents oneself socially. Sexual orientation is defined as emotional, romantic, and sexual attraction to one, multiple, all, or no sexes/genders.

The first step in assessing eligibility for a medical intervention is gaining a better understanding of the youth's understanding of their sex, gender, and gender expression. This is best accomplished with careful assessment by a mental health professional with experience in working with youth around topics of gender. Important considerations to explore include the following: When did the child or adolescent begin considering gender in more detail? How is the youth experiencing pubertal changes? Are pubertal changes causing distress or anxiety? What is the youth's current understanding of how medical interventions work, and what would they expect to happen to their bodies if medical interventions are used? How do their parents perceive their gender identity now and historically? What is the level of support for gender exploration in the youth's home and in the youth's community? Are there co-occurring mental health comorbidities present such as anxiety and depression and are these comorbidities in reasonable control? Does the child meet Diagnostic and Statistical Manual of Mental Disorders, 5th edition, criteria for gender dysphoria?

Regardless of the answers to these questions, there is little in the medical literature and clinical guidelines around endocrine treatment for the gender-expansive or gender nonbinary youth. The original utility of using GnRH agonists was, in essence, to buy time for the adolescent to make a balanced decision about gender without the stress of the progression of dysphoric puberty. We would argue that gender-expansive, genderqueer, or gender nonbinary youth would not be good candidates for GnRH agonists unless there is dysphoria related to the current progression, or the anticipated progression of isosexual puberty. If a GnRH agonist was felt to be appropriate for an individual under these circumstances, indefinite suppression of puberty without endogenous puberty or exogenous sex steroid treatment is not recommended.

Financial Considerations

Guidelines are only theoretical if they recommend treatments that are unavailable. GnRH agonist medications are extremely expensive and not affordable to most families if not covered by medical insurance. While providers in various geographical locations have had different success with respect to coverage, it is clear that access to GnRH agonist treatment is not universal.[14] Barriers to universal coverage of GnRH agonist treatment for transgender youth may include (1) it is not Food and Drug Administration approved for use outside of treatment for youth with precocious puberty, (2) long-term data on safety and efficacy is deemed not robust by some, and (3) gender-affirming treatment is not mandated for coverage in all areas. Approval or denial of GnRH agonist treatment has serious practical implications for the individual patient and may significantly impact the care plan.

For a child in early puberty, who is eligible for, but cannot afford GnRH agonist treatment, limited options exist. One consideration would be exploration of different formulations of GnRH agonists. For example, the GnRH agonist designed for use in adults with prostate cancer (Vantas, Endo Pharmaceuticals) is much less expensive than the formulation used in children with precocious puberty (Supprelin, Endo Pharmaceuticals).[14] Additionally, treatment of transgender youth with medroxyprogesterone to suppress puberty has also been described.[39] Lastly, and concerningly, the adolescent who would otherwise be started on GnRH agonist treatment to delay pubertal decisions regarding sex steroid therapy, but who cannot afford the blocker, may prompt more urgent discussion about readiness for initiation of gender-affirming hormones.

INITIATION OF GENDER-AFFIRMING HORMONES

Gender-affirming hormones, testosterone and estrogen, are used to promote development of secondary sex characteristics aligned with a person's gender identity. As discussed above, age of initiation is a topic of ongoing conversation in the field of transgender medicine. Historically, 16 years of age was used in the "Dutch Protocol" as this is the age of consent in the Netherlands. This historical tradition was carried forward in the WPATH SOC and the Endocrine Society Guidelines. That said, the revised version of the Endocrine Society Guidelines (2017) notes that delaying treatment with these hormones until 16 years of age may not be in the best interest for all patients.[7] In order to assess this historical practice, we should consider the risks and benefits of delaying treatment.

Perhaps the original impetus for delaying treatment to 16 years of age in the Netherlands was to allow for legal consent for treatment. However, this rationale only applies to the Netherlands or other countries where the age of medical consent is 16 years. If the same rationale were applied to the United States, perhaps patients would need to wait until 18 years of age to consent for testosterone or estrogen. It is important to note that delaying puberty until the age of 16 years is not physiologic. Thus, waiting to begin puberty until the age of 18 years would alter the normal timing of puberty to an even more dramatic extent and is not a practical course of treatment. Furthermore, there is concern that the longer an adolescent remains prepubertal on GnRH analog suppression, the higher the risk for low bone mineral density. Finally, withholding pubertal hormones until the age of 16 years may be socially and emotionally difficult for an adolescent, making pubertal timing delayed compared to their peers.

In his description of endocrine considerations for transgender youth, Rosenthal notes that at the time of writing (2014), his institution (UCSF) was studying the impact of cross-sex hormone treatment at the age of 14 years, which is an age similar to the upper end of normal pubertal onset.[37]

An alternative approach considers patient and family readiness, rather than any particular age cutoff, as the most important factor for the initiation of gender-affirming hormones. This approach would allow for initiation of testosterone or estrogen at any age after pubertal onset. This approach takes into account the fact that a 12-year-old on a GnRH agonist since the age of 9 years, who perhaps made a social transition at the age of 6 years, may be a better candidate for testosterone or estrogen than a 15-year-old who is in the early stages of exploring their gender identity.

Ultimately, it is our opinion that arbitrary age cutoffs are not particularly helpful on the individual level and that an individualized approach is preferred based on patient readiness, assessed by a mental health professional with expertise in gender identity. However, prior to the accrual of long-term data, providers should be cautious when starting gender-affirming hormones in early adolescence.

TESTOSTERONE

Transgender men and boys are prescribed testosterone to promote development of male secondary sex characteristics. Testosterone is most often prescribed as an intramuscular or subcutaneous injection (testosterone cypionate or testosterone enanthate) once weekly or once every 2 weeks. The adult dose of injectable testosterone is typically 50–100 mg/week or 100–200 mg/2 weeks. When treating transgender boys who have been treated with GnRH agonists, or even adolescents who have not been on GnRH agonists, the goal is to mimic normal puberty, which begins gradually. Therefore, dosing often starts lower, perhaps at 12.5 mg/week or 25 mg/2 weeks, and increases over time to the adult dose.[37] Titration of dosing is based on the development of desired masculinizing effects, suppression of menses if not co-treated with a GnRH agonist, and monitoring of testosterone levels with a goal of an age-appropriate male testosterone level.

Alternative formulations of testosterone include transdermal patches or testosterone gel. These formulations are most often prescribed once the full adult dose has been reached using injectable testosterone; however, these can also be considered in the patient with needle phobia.[37] Testosterone treatment likely increases the risk of polycythemia, sleep apnea, weight gain, and cystic acne and possibly increases the risk of elevated liver enzymes, hyperlipidemia, and hypertension.[6]

ESTROGEN

Transgender girls and women are treated with estrogen in order to achieve feminine secondary sex characteristics. 17-β-estradiol is the preferred formulation of estrogen and is available as a transdermal patch, oral tablet, or as an injectable. In pediatric patients, transdermal patches and oral tablets are most commonly prescribed. The dosing of estrogen, as described above, varies depending on co-treatment with a GnRH agonist. The required dose of 17-β-estradiol is much lower for the suppressed patient. For the suppressed transgender woman, the typical adult dose of 17-β-estradiol is typically 2 mg when given as an oral tablet, and 0.1 mg/ 24 h patch when given as a transdermal patch. However, when not suppressed, the required dose may be as high as 6–8 mg orally, or 0.4 mg/24 h transdermal patch.[22] Similarly to testosterone, younger patients on GnRH agonist treatment typically start at lower doses and gradually increase to the adult dose. Titration of dosing is based on the development of desired feminizing effects, suppression of testosterone effects such as erections and facial/body hair development, and testosterone and estrogen levels in the age-appropriate female range.[37] Estrogen treatment likely increases the risk of thromboembolic disease (particularly synthetic ethinyl estradiol), hypertriglyceridemia, gallstones, elevated liver enzymes, and weight gain and may increase the risk of hypertension and hyperprolactinemia.[6]

CONCLUSIONS

The field of transgender medicine is growing, and arguably maturing from its infancy into its adolescence. Endocrine treatment of transgender youth began with the observation that earlier treatment, including pubertal blockade, could provide significant reduction in dysphoria in adolescence and improved physical and mental health outcomes. As these observations became Guidelines and SOC, logistical and safety questions emerged, which have not been fully resolved. While current guidelines provide a framework for treatment, they fail to address important questions that commonly arise in clinical care. It is our hope that this chapter fills some of these gaps. Clearly, further research is needed to inform best practices in the care of the transgender adolescent. Simultaneously, financial barriers to care must be addressed in order for all transgender youth to receive access to gender-affirming treatment.

REFERENCES

1. Shumer DE, Spack NP. Current management of gender identity disorder in childhood and adolescence: guidelines, barriers and areas of controversy. *Curr Opin Endocrinol Diabetes Obes.* 2013;20(1):69–73. https://doi.org/10.1097/MED.0b013e32835c711e.
2. American Psychiatric Association. *Diagnostic and Statistical Manual of Mental Disorders.* 5th ed. 2013.
3. Delemarre-Van de Waal HA, Cohen-Kettenis PT. Clinical management of gender identity disorder in adolescents: a protocol on psychological and paediatric endocrinology aspects. *Eur J Endocrinol.* 2006;155(suppl 1):S131–S137. https://doi.org/10.1530/eje.1.02231.
4. Carel J, Léger J. Precocious puberty. *N Engl J Med.* 2008; 358(22):2366–2377.
5. Kaplowitz PB. Delayed puberty. *Pediatr Rev.* 2010;31(5): 189–195. https://doi.org/10.1542/pir.31-5-189.
6. Coleman E, Bockting W, Botzer M, et al. Standards of care for the health of transsexual, transgender, and gender-nonconforming People, version 7. *Int J Transgend.* 2012;13(4):165–232. https://doi.org/10.1080/15532739.2011.700873.
7. Hembree WC, Cohen-Kettenis PT, Gooren L, et al. Endocrine treatment of gender-dysphoric/gender-incongruent persons: an endocrine society* clinical practice guideline. *J Clin Endocrinol Metab.* 2017;102(11):1–35. https://doi.org/10.1210/jc.2017-01658.
8. Edwards-Leeper L, Spack NP. Psychological evaluation and medical treatment of transgender youth in an interdisciplinary "Gender Management Service" (GeMS) in a major pediatric center. *J Homosex.* 2012;59(3):321–336. https://doi.org/10.1080/00918369.2012.653302.
9. Eliason MJ, Streed CG. Choosing "Something Else" as a sexual identity: evaluating response options on the national health interview survey. *LGBT Health.* 2017; 4(5):376–379. https://doi.org/10.1089/lgbt.2016.0206.
10. Zucker KJ, Lawrence AA. Epidemiology of gender identity disorder: recommendations for the standards of care of the World Professional Association for transgender health. *Int J Transgend.* 2009;11(1):8–18. https://doi.org/10.1080/15532730902799946.
11. Conron K, Scott G, Stowell G, Landers S. Transgender health in Massachusetts: results from a household probability sample of adults. *Am J Public Health.* 2012;102:118–122.
12. Crissman HP, Berger MB, Graham LF, Dalton VK. Transgender demographics: a household probability sample of US adults, 2014. *Am J Public Health.* 2017;107(2): 213–215. https://doi.org/10.2105/AJPH.2016.303571.
13. Flores AR, Herman JL, Gates GJ, Brown TNT. How many adults identify as transgender in the United States? *The Williams Institue.* 2016;(June):13.
14. Stevens J, Gomez-Lobo V, Pine-Twaddell E. Insurance coverage of puberty blocker therapies for transgender youth. *Pediatrics.* 2015;136(6):1029–1031.
15. Marcell AV. Adolescence. In: Kligman RM, Behrman RE, Jenson HB, Stanton BF, eds. *Nelson Textbook of Pediatrics.* 18th ed. Philadelphia: Saunders Elsevier; 2007:60–65.
16. Fuqua JS. Treatment and outcomes of precocious puberty: an update. *J Clin Endocrinol Metab.* 2013;98(6): 2198–2207. https://doi.org/10.1210/jc.2013-1024.
17. Rosenfield RL, Cooke DW, Radovick S. Development of the female reproductive system. In: Sperling MA, ed. *Pediatric Endocrinology.* 3rd ed. Philadelphia: Saunders Elsevier; 2008:532–559.
18. Cohen-Kettenis PT, Klink D. Adolescents with gender dysphoria. *Best Pract Res Clin Endocrinol Metab.* 2015;29(3): 485–495. https://doi.org/10.1016/j.beem.2015.01.004.
19. Vrouenraets LJJJ, Fredriks AM, Hannema SE, Cohen-Kettenis PT, de Vries MC. Perceptions of sex, gender, and puberty suppression: a qualitative analysis of transgender youth. *Arch Sex Behav.* 2016;45(7):1697–1703. https://doi.org/10.1007/s10508-016-0764-9.

20. Cohen-Kettenis PT, Delemarre-van De Waal HA, Gooren LJG. The treatment of adolescent transsexuals: changing insights. *J Sex Med.* 2008;5(8):1892−1897. https://doi.org/10.1111/j.1743-6109.2008.00870.x.

21. De Vries ALC, Cohen-Kettenis PT. Clinical management of gender dysphoria in children and adolescents: the Dutch approach. *J Homosex.* 2012;59(3):301−320. https://doi.org/10.1080/00918369.2012.653300.

22. Center of Excellence for Transgender Health, Department of Family, Community Medicine, Univesity of California San Francisco. In: Deutsch MB, ed. *Guidelines for the Primary and Gender-affirming Care of Transgender and Gender Nonbinary People.* 2nd ed. 2016. Available from: www.transhealth.ucsf.edu/guidelines.

23. Biro FM, Galvez MP, Greenspan LC, et al. Pubertal assessment method and baseline characteristics in a mixed longitudinal study of girls. *Pediatrics.* 2010;126(3): e583−e590. https://doi.org/10.1542/peds.2009-3079.

24. De Vries ALC, Steensma TD, Doreleijers TA, Cohen-Kettenis PT. Puberty suppression in adolescents with gender identity disorder: a prospective follow-up study. *J Sex Med.* 2011;8:2276−2283.

25. Steensma TD, McGuire JK, Kreukels BPC, Beekman AJ, Cohen-Kettenis PT. Factors associated with desistence and persistence of childhood gender dysphoria: a quantitative follow-up study. *J Am Acad Child Adolesc Psychiatry.* 2013; 52(6):582−590. https://doi.org/10.1016/j.jaac.2013.03.016.

26. Schagen SEE, Cohen-Kettenis PT, Delemarre-van de Waal HA, Hannema SE. Efficacy and safety of gonadotropin-releasing hormone agonist treatment to suppress puberty in gender dysphoric adolescents. *J Sex Med.* 2016;13(7):1125−1132. https://doi.org/10.1016/j.jsxm.2016.05.004.

27. Parent A-S, Teilmann G, Juul A, Skakkebaek NE, Toparri J, Bourguignon J-P. The timing of normal puberty and the age limits of sexual precocity: variations around the World, secular trends, and changes after migration. *Endocr Rev.* 2003;24(5):668−693. https://doi.org/10.1210/er.2002-0019.

28. Berberoğlu M. Precocious puberty and normal variant puberty: definition, etiology, diagnosis and current management. *J Clin Res Pediatr Endocrinol.* 2009;1(4): 164−174. https://doi.org/10.4274/jcrpe.v1i4.3.

29. Palmert MR, Dunkel L. Delayed puberty. *N Engl J Med.* 2012;366:443−453.

30. Klink D, Caris M, Heijboer A, van Trotsenburg M, Rotteveel J. Bone mass in young adulthood following gonadotropin-releasing hormone analog treatment and cross-sex hormone treatment in adolescents with gender dysphoria. *J Clin Endocrinol Metab.* 2015;100(2): E270−E275. https://doi.org/10.1210/jc.2014-2439.

31. Donnez J, Dolmans M-M. Fertility preservation in women. *N Engl J Med.* 2017;377(17):1657−1665. https://doi.org/10.1056/NEJMra1614676.

32. Light AD, Obedin-Maliver J, Sevelius JM, Kerns JL. Transgender men who experienced pregnancy after female-to-male gender transitioning. *Obstet Gynecol.* 2014;124(6):1120−1127. https://doi.org/10.1097/AOG.0000000000000540.

33. Klink D, Bokenkamp A, Dekker C, Rotteveel J. Arterial hypertension as a complication of Triptorelin treatment in adolescents with gender dysphoria. *Endocrinol Metab Int J.* 2015;2(1):8−11. https://doi.org/10.15406/emij.2015.02.00008.

34. Sørensen K, Aksglaede L, Petersen JH, Juul A. Recent changes in pubertal timing in healthy Danish boys: associations with body mass index. *J Clin Endocrinol Metab.* 2010;95(1):263−270. https://doi.org/10.1210/jc.2009-1478.

35. Herman-Giddens ME, Steffes J, Harris D, et al. Secondary sexual characteristics in boys: data from the pediatric research in office settings network. *Pediatrics.* 2012;130(5): e1058−e1068. https://doi.org/10.1542/peds.2011-3291.

36. Ramaswamy S, Weinbauer GF. Endocrine control of spermatogenesis: role of FSH and LH/testosterone. *Spermatogenesis.* 2014;4(2).

37. Rosenthal SM. Approach to the patient: transgender youth: endocrine considerations. *J Clin Endocrinol Metab.* 2014; 99(12):4379−4389.

38. Gooren PhD LJ. Care of transsexual persons. *N Engl J Med.* 2011;364:1251−1257.

39. Lynch MM, Khandheria MM, Meyer WJ. Retrospective study of the management of childhood and adolescent gender identity disorder using medroxyprogesterone acetate. *Int J Transgend.* 2015;16(4):201−208.

CHAPTER 11

Ethical Considerations of GnRHa Treatment and Consent Process

REBECCA M. HARRIS, MD, PHD, MA • JOEL E. FRADER, MD, MA

INTRODUCTION

Over the last decade, the medical treatment of transgender youth has evolved. In medicine and in much of Western society, there is a movement to acknowledge that biological sex and gender identity are distinct entities. Furthermore, many now challenge the idea that gender identity only involves a binary male/female system; numerous individuals believe gender identity is fluid and can occur along a spectrum.[1]

At this time, we lack precise data regarding how many children and young adults identify as transgender. Extrapolating from studies of adults, the prevalence may be as high as 1 in 200.[2,3] Multidisciplinary clinics for transgender youth have experienced an increase in patient enrollment over the last several years.[1] Additionally, the number of younger children presenting to clinics for gender nonconforming youth has increased. The rising number of patients presenting to gender clinics and the younger age at presentation likely result from a combination of factors, including (1) increased access to information from the Internet, (2) more media and other public attention to transgender individuals in society, and (3) increased openness between parents and educational and healthcare professionals about gender nonconforming behavior.[4] While there is no "typical age" at which recognition of gender incongruence occurs, a recent study found the average age was 8.3 years. The standard deviation found in the research study was 4.5 years, indicating children younger than 4 years experienced gender incongruence.[5]

Multiple factors complicate the medical management of transgender youth. First, transgender youth have high rates of depression, suicidal ideation, and self-harm compared to non-LGBT (lesbian, gay, bisexual, transgender) peers.[6] In one study, 35% of transgender youth had depression, more than 50% had suicidal ideation, and 33% had attempted suicide.[5] Therefore, clinicians have an obligation to identify and secure treatment for these serious mental health conditions, in addition to addressing any gender dysphoria. Also confounding initiation of specific medical management of transgender youth is the elusive ability to predict which children will "persist" and remain transgender and which children will "desist" and find congruence with their natal sex.

In this chapter, we discuss the ethical issues involved in pubertal suppression of transgender youth. We first provide background information on current methods of pubertal suppression, the known effects of gonadotropin-releasing hormone (GnRH) agonists, and the benefits of pubertal suppression. We explore the ethical issues involved in pubertal suppression with GnRH agonists in transgender youth, looking at beneficence, nonmaleficence, autonomy, and informed consent and assent. The ethical issues involving gender-affirming hormones (GAHs) and gender-affirming surgery, while interesting, are beyond the scope of this chapter.

PUBERTAL SUPPRESSION

Physiologically, pubertal progression begins with GnRH pulses from the hypothalamus. This results in production of gonadotropins, luteinizing hormone and follicle stimulating hormone, from the pituitary. The gonadotropins then stimulate the gonads to produce sex hormones, namely testosterone in natal males and estrogen in natal females. Clinically, the first sign of puberty in girls is thelarche, with development of breast tissue. On average, thelarche occurs between the ages of 8 and 13 years. In boys, the first sign of puberty is testicular enlargement. In natal males, secondary sex characteristics typically appear between the ages of 9 and 14 years. The five-point Tanner staging system denotes progression of physical changes through puberty. Tanner stage 1 is prepubertal and Tanner stage 5 signifies full pubertal development.[7]

Clinical pubertal suppression involves administration of GnRH agonists. The lay term for GnRH agonists is "blockers" as they "block" puberty. Treatment with a GnRH agonist results in tonic, rather than pulsatile levels of GnRH. Without pulsatile GnRH, the hypothalamic–pituitary–gonadal axis is suppressed. With this suppression, the amount of sex hormone (testosterone in natal males and estrogen in natal females) produced by the gonads decreases and pubertal progression stops.[7] In the United States, clinicians use two GnRH agonists, leuprolide (brand name Lupron) and histrelin (brand name Supprelin). Leuprolide, an injectable GnRH agonist is administered once a month or once every 3 months. Histrelin, an implant placed subcutaneously, delivers medication for up to 2 years. Histrelin can be implanted with or without sedation.[4]

Pubertal suppression with GnRH agonists first saw clinical use in patients with precocious puberty to stop pubertal progression and provide additional time for the child to grow.[8] In 2006, a group in the Netherlands created a protocol for the use of GnRH agonists in transgender patients as young as 12 years.[9] The goal was to suppress puberty in order to treat gender dysphoria.[4] In 2009, the Endocrine Society, along with the World Professional Association for Transgender Health and several other organizations, created a clinical practice guideline recommending the use of GnRH agonists for pubertal suppression in transgender children. However, instead of stipulating an age for initiating the use of GnRH agonists, the guidelines recommended their use as early as Tanner 2, which can occur before 12 years of age.[10] The Endocrine Society also recommended psychological assessments of patients to ascertain their readiness for treatment and ensure that mental health comorbidities be addressed along with gender dysphoria. The guidelines further recommended ongoing patient follow-up by a mental health provider throughout medical treatment.[10]

Currently, GnRH agonists are the standard of care for pubertal suppression in transgender youth.[4] Clinicians generally believe that blocking puberty with GnRH agonists is fully reversible. However, there are limited safety and efficacy studies, and medical science has virtually no data on the safety or effectiveness of GnRH agonists in transgender children younger than 12 years.[1]

GnRH agonists do have known side effects. Approximately a month after the initial administration, a surge of sex hormones, testosterone in natal males and estrogen in natal females, can occur, resulting in acceleration of natal puberty or even initiation of menstruation, with substantial distress for the patient. An additional leuprolide injection 2 weeks after the initial injection or implant insertion counteracts these side effects. Local site reactions (i.e., pain, swelling, abscess), rash, hot flushes, and sweating can all occur, as well.[4]

BENEFITS OF PUBERTAL SUPPRESSION

Pubertal suppression with GnRH agonists constitutes the first step in the medical treatment of transgender youth with gender dysphoria.[4] GnRH agonists provide several benefits to trans-youth. First and foremost, GnRH agonists prevent the development of natal secondary sex characteristics, which cause substantial emotional turmoil in transgender patients, worsening dysphoria and exacerbating psychiatric comorbidities.[5] Additionally, postponing the "wrong" puberty, can allow the patient to focus more fully on mental health therapy.[4] Second, delaying puberty provides transgender youth and their families time to think about their needs and goals before deciding whether to continue with more "permanent" aspects of the gender transition process.[4,11] While patients have sometimes had ample time to think through their circumstances and aspirations, it often takes family members longer to understand the situation, see things from the patient's perspective, and accept a radical change in their expectations and hopes for their child. Families also often need time to learn about the benefits and risks of medical treatment. Third, if the child and the family decide to continue with the gender transition, preventing natal secondary sex characteristics allows for optimal transition.[12] Preventing the formation of natal secondary sex characteristics by halting natal puberty can reduce or eliminate the need for surgeries that reverse or ameliorate the secondary sex characteristics (developed breasts, Adam's apple, facial bone development in natal males, and so on).[4] Those surgeries and accompanying anesthesia have inherent risks, and preventing the need for surgery eliminates those hazards.

ETHICAL ISSUES
Research

Research focusing on transgender youth has been limited, though it is starting to expand.[12] Only over the last decade have investigations into the effects of the medical treatment of transgender youth occurred.

The majority of clinical recommendations were based on expert opinion or data from the adult transgender population, neither of which is ideal.[1] While expert opinion may be useful in rare diseases that are difficult to study, anecdotal evidence is often biased. Extrapolating from adult data to pediatric populations also has significant flaws. Most importantly, children are indeed not small adults, physiologically or emotionally. The changes that occur during childhood and adolescence do not continue into adulthood. Studying medication effects during adulthood does not take those developmental variables into account. The use of GnRH agonists to prevent puberty likely has effects on the child-to-adult developmental processes that knowledge based on their use in adults cannot anticipate.

Additionally, the majority of adult studies in the literature are observational and thus have distinct biases. Often observational research relies on accounts of previous events; subjects can have recall bias and may be unable to accurately recount the past. Additionally, societal norms and structures change quickly, and what was true for a subject a decade ago may no longer have relevance for individuals now. Finally, developmental differences exist in how children and adults make decisions, and analyses based on adult decision-making do not take those differences into account. The lack of high quality research in the trans-youth population has prompted an interest in developing evidence-based clinical practice in pediatric transgender patients. The first multicentered, National Institutes of Health–funded study in the United States investigating the impact of psychosocial factors and medical treatment on transgender youth began enrolling subjects in 2016.[13]

Multiple factors have contributed to the lack of research in transgender youth. First, children are considered a vulnerable class, and numerous ethical and regulatory constraints limit research in these populations, though exceptions may apply.[14,15] Transgender youth younger than 18 years in the United States are vulnerable simply based on age, though their high rate of mental and sexual health comorbidities certainly create emotional vulnerability as well. There is a history of unethical research in vulnerable populations, which decades ago resulted in more strict ethical guidelines for the conduct of research, especially in these populations.[16] Researchers and institutional review boards (IRBs) must now exercise considerable caution regarding the potential for coercion, particularly in situations where few, if any, satisfactory clinical options exist. As a result, researchers may anticipate or have difficulty obtaining IRB approval for studies involving transgender youth and may hesitate to propose studies that include this population. However, this reluctance exacerbates the problem by perpetuating the lack of treatment with proven effectiveness. It also creates a vicious cycle: LGBT adolescents continue to have inadequate sexual and mental healthcare compared to their peers, and the lack of research prevents progress in addressing these disparities.[17] This exemplifies the need for ethically conducted research in vulnerable populations.

The relative low incidence and/or prevalence of conditions also creates challenges for conducting high-quality research.[12] Researchers need to meet or exceed threshold numbers of subjects to sufficiently power studies. Individual medical centers may not have adequate potential subjects to undertake statistically valid research. While multicenter trials can provide more subjects to achieve adequate statistical power, the logistics of coordinating trials across multiple centers and finding funding for such studies create formidable obstacles.

Additionally, researchers, regulators, and ethicists debate what kinds of studies are ethically permissible. Most contend that randomized control trials (RCTs) provide the greatest rigor and yield the most reliable clinical information. In RCTs, subjects are randomly assigned to an unproven treatment arm, to a placebo arm, or to a conventional (standard care) arm, if applicable. Most stakeholders agree that for transgender youth, it would be morally unacceptable to provide GnRH agonists to some subjects and placebos to others, thus denying any treatment, in order to study the short- and long-term effects of hormone blockers.[12]

Additionally, experience gained with GnRH agonists in other contexts suggests that the harms are likely not great, making a placebo arm unnecessary or simply wrong. However, some clinicians and researchers would argue that the information about the harm of GnRH blockade is circumstantial and has the potential to be so great that it is morally wrong not to conduct a placebo-controlled trial.

Balancing Beneficence and Nonmaleficence

Beneficence and nonmaleficence are core ethical principles in medicine. Beneficence is the desire to do good. Nonmaleficence is the desire to do no harm.[18] The challenge lies in balancing doing good while also avoiding inadvertent or unknowable harm. In the trans-youth population, one way for physicians to "do good" is to treat gender dysphoria with GnRH agonists,

GAHs, and gender-affirming surgery. However, treatment of gender dysphoria with medications not yet fully proven safe and effective in trans-youth involves unknown risks. While GnRH agonists in children with precocious puberty effectively halt puberty progression, that fact alone does not establish that these drugs relieve symptoms of gender dysphoria.[19] At this time, there are limited data about the psychological impact of GnRH agonists. There is one study from 2014 by a group in the Netherlands evaluating the psychosocial impact of GnRH agonists, GAHs, and surgery in trans-youth. Gender dysphoria and body image dissatisfaction persisted through puberty blockade with GnRH agonists but were relieved after GAHs and surgery.[19] This is not surprising as GnRH agonists simply halt pubertal progression but do not result in development of secondary sex characteristics of the affirmed gender. However, their use in conjunction with GAHs and gender-affirming surgery has been shown to improve gender dysphoria.[19]

The long-term effects of GnRH agonists on bone formation, cognitive development, and future fertility are also unknown.[1] In terms of bone health, sex steroids promote bone growth and mineralization.[7] Pubertal suppression with GnRH agonists results in decreased production of natal sex steroids during the period of suppression. Therefore, the use of GnRH agonists could negatively impact bone density. Additionally, as trans-youth may now receive treatment before Tanner 2, this creates a population of children exposed to long courses of GnRH agonists, extending the period of low sex steroids.

The use of GnRH agonists in children with precocious puberty does not impair bone mass or final height.[20] However, trans-youth differ from individuals with precocious puberty in that the latter have already been exposed to pubertal sex steroids while young transgender children may have had very limited exposure. A longitudinal observational study from the Netherlands published in 2015 showed that trans-youth who had undergone pubertal suppression with GnRH agonists and treatment with GAHs had decreased bone mineral density compared to pretreatment bone density. The researchers concluded that either peak bone mass was delayed or attenuated. However, the study had several limitations. The subject pool was not robust ($n = 34$). The exact cause of the decreased bone mass was unknown and confounded by variations in the duration of GnRH agonist treatment, low initial GAH dosing, and other factors, including the use of GAHs. Many of the subjects had already started puberty and thus already had some exposure to endogenous natal sex steroids, which could affect the results. The duration of GnRH agonist therapy was often brief. Also, the published study provided no information about diet and exercise, which contribute to bone density.[21] Taken together, these limitations highlight the need for additional research.

Another topic in trans-youth healthcare that entails ethical issues and requires additional research concerns fertility preservation. Current methods of fertility preservation include sperm freezing for postpubertal males and oocyte cryopreservation for postpubertal females. For prepubertal individuals, fertility preservation techniques are still experimental. If prepubertal trans-youth on GnRH agonists want to preserve oocytes or sperm, clinical protocols require them to stop the GnRH agonist and proceed through natal puberty in order to harvest gametes, which can be extremely distressing for the transgender individual.[4] In the future, it may be possible to cryopreserve prepubertal gonadal tissue and mature the gametes in vitro, however at this time prepubertal gonadal cryopreservation remains experimental.[22]

To date, no studies have appeared in the medical literature on the isolated impact of GnRH agonists on future reproductive ability in transgender youth. The belief that GnRH agonists do not affect future fertility comes from inferences based on studies in patients with central precocious puberty (CPP).[23] Isolating the reproductive effects of GnRH agonists in individuals with CPP presents fewer challenges than assessing the situation in transgender individuals, as the latter typically have also received GAHs, confounding the effects of GnRH agonists alone on fertility. It does not seem possible to investigate and isolate the impact of GnRH agonists on the future reproductive potential of trans-youth. It does seem imperative to study the impact medical treatment as a whole (GnRH agonists and GAHs) may have on future reproductive potential of transgender individuals.

Research thus far has focused on the use of fertility preservation in the trans-youth population. In 2017, a retrospective review of 73 trans-youth patients showed that 72 had fertility counseling prior to GAHs and only two subjects attempted fertility preservation (both natal males). Of the subjects, 45% discussed adopting and 21% did not want children.[24]

Many reasons might lead the majority of trans-youth offered fertility preservation to decline. Children and adolescents may not be developmentally ready to make decisions about their future fertility. Additionally, trans-youth often feel a sense of urgency with gender transitioning and are thus not willing to delay treatment (with GAHs) to harvest sperm or eggs.[12] For some trans-youth who may want biological children in the future, the idea of using natal eggs or sperm that do not align with their gender identity seems too discordant.[25] Other barriers to fertility preservation exist: cost, insurance coverage, invasiveness of the procedures, potential societal pressure about what comprises a "nuclear" family, and objections by parents, other family members, or romantic partners.

Nevertheless, perspectives often change with age and maturity, and once transgender children reach adulthood, they may regret no longer having the ability to produce biological children because they did not preserve eggs or sperm. Data from transgender adults have been mixed, with some studies showing transgender adults would have considered fertility preservation if the option had been available and other studies showing relatively little desire for biological children.[26–28] Unfortunately, transgender individuals may encounter difficulty adopting, as reports have appeared recounting challenges for transgender individuals in achieving approval to become adoptive parents.[24] For the above reasons, it is important to (1) understand the impact of the medical treatment of transgender youth on future fertility and (2) discuss with the patient and family all of the potential options for future fertility before irreversible medical treatment occurs.

Respect for Autonomy: Assent and Consent

The ethical principle of autonomy refers to the ability of individuals to make their own decisions.[18] This concept is more complicated in pediatrics as patients typically have not yet reached the age of majority, become statutorily emancipated, or received judicial determination as mature minors and therefore cannot legally authorize their own treatment or provide consent. Instead, minor children are asked to provide assent and the patient's guardian, typically a parent, must provide consent. Regardless of legal status, engaging the patient in medical decision-making constitutes an ethical cornerstone of care for all youth. Clinicians must discuss medical issues with patients using developmentally appropriate language, taking into account the patient's cognitive abilities and maturity. Maturity, of course, does not always correlate with age; young and mature individuals can and should participate more fully in medical decision-making than older patients who lack maturity or cognitive ability.[29]

In the trans-youth population, the concept of autonomy has particular relevance and complexity. Children now present to gender clinics at younger ages than even in recent years, and medicine has no definitive means to identify which children will "persist" along the transgender path and which children will "desist" and continue along the course of their natal sex. Some data suggest that two factors correlate with persistence of transgender identity: greater gender dysphoria and being a natal female. Of course, these attributes do not predict what will occur for each patient.[30] The inability to know which patients will complete the gender transition creates difficulty in balancing the child's interest in making autonomous choices and desire for immediate medical treatment with the goals of beneficence and nonmaleficence.[30,31] Medical professionals understandably hesitate to initiate irreversible treatments knowing the patient may later view the treatment as unnecessary and regrettable.[12]

In addition, patients and parents/guardians may have discordant perspectives on transgender treatment. Trans-youth below the age of 18 years and not emancipated need guardian consent to proceed with medical treatment. Guardians who support the child's gender identity may provide consent for medical treatment with GnRH agonists and GAHs. However, for patients whose guardians are reluctant or slow to accept their gender identity or who reject the child's feelings and choices and therefore will not provide consent, medical treatment can be delayed. The postponement of medical care can impose extreme distress on the transgender child or adolescent. In cases of guardian refusal to provide consent, the patient may have to wait until the age of 18 years to start medical treatment, which means that patient will undergo full pubertal progression and will acquire secondary sexual characteristics of the wrong gender.[12] In cases where parents share guardianship and one parent accepts treatment but the other parent does not, treatment may also be delayed until both guardians can agree or the patient reaches the age of majority.

Further, the very notion of fully informed consent for transgender treatment can prove problematic. The patient and guardian can only learn what medical information is known. Where clinicians have limited understanding of the long-term effects of medications, full informed consent seems impossible to achieve. Professionals must clearly explain what they know and do not know and the potential long-term effects of available treatments. Families may find the uncertainty very difficult to grasp and/or accept, leading to unwillingness to proceed.

CONCLUSION

Pubertal suppression for transgender youth presents a multiple of ethically complex issues. The lack of knowledge about the long-term impact of GnRH agonists on transgender youth makes providing full informed consent and assent problematic with the unknown risks of long-term treatment undermining meaningful exercise of patient autonomy. The uncertainty also limits medical professionals' attempts to balance beneficence and nonmaleficence in counseling patients and families.

However, it would be inappropriate and unrealistic to stop using GnRH agonists to suppress pubertal development in children with gender dysphoria while we wait for more data. Having these children progress through a natal puberty would cause great emotional distress for many patients and makes later treatment, especially surgery, more difficult and less effective. Thus, refusal to use hormone blockade goes against the principle of nonmaleficence and would, in fact, impose harm. Despite the limited data about the positive psychological impact of GnRH agonists alone, we endorse the use of GnRH agonists due to the benefit of preventing natal secondary sex characteristics and providing time for patients and families to decide the best course of action.[19] While GnRH agonists alone may not improve gender dysphoria, they constitute a vital part of the protocol for treatment of gender dysphoria.

To address the ethical issues in the medical care of trans-youth, the affected population and those that provide treatment need additional research about the long-term effects of treatment. Only such evidence will permit medical professionals to act in a beneficent manner and enable patients and families to adequately exercise autonomous decision-making. For now, clear communication with patients and their families must include acknowledgement of the limits of medical knowledge regarding the offered treatment in order to promote autonomy in consent and assent.

REFERENCES

1. Rosenthal SM. Transgender youth: current concepts. *Ann Pediatr Endocrinol Metab.* 2016;21421:185−192. https://doi.org/10.6065/apem.2016.21.4.185.
2. Conron KJ, Scott G, Stowell GS, Landers SJ. Transgender health in Massachusetts: results from a household probability sample of adults. *Am J Public Health.* 2012;102(1):118−122. https://doi.org/10.2105/AJPH.2011.300315.
3. Crissman HP, Berger MB, Graham LF, Dalton VK. Transgender demographics: a household probability sample of US adults, 2014. *Am J Public Health.* 2017;107(2):213−215. https://doi.org/10.2105/AJPH.2016.303571.
4. Olson J, Garofalo R. The peripubertal gender-dysphoric child: puberty suppression and treatment paradigms. *Pediatr Ann.* 2014;43(6):e132−e137. https://doi.org/10.3928/00904481-20140522-08.
5. Olson J, Schrager SM, Belzer M, Simons LK, Clark LF. Baseline physiologic and psychosocial characteristics of transgender youth seeking care for gender dysphoria. *J Adolesc Health.* 2015;57(4):374−380. https://doi.org/10.1016/j.jadohealth.2015.04.027.
6. Almeida J, Johnson RM, Corliss HL, Molnar BE, Azrael D. Emotional distress among LGBT youth: the influence of perceived discrimination based on sexual orientation. *J Youth Adolesc.* 2009;38(7):1001−1014. https://doi.org/10.1007/s10964-009-9397-9.
7. Sperling MA. *Pediatric Endocrinology.* 4th ed. Elsevier; 2014.
8. Carel J-C, Eugster EA, Rogol A, Ghizzoni L, Palmert MR. Consensus statement on the use of gonadotropin-releasing hormone analogs in children. *Pediatrics.* 2009;123(4):e752−e762. https://doi.org/10.1542/peds.2008-1783.
9. Delemarre-van de Waal HA, Cohen-Kettenis PT. Clinical management of gender identity disorder in adolescents: a protocol on psychological and paediatric endocrinology aspects. *Eur J Endocrinol.* 2006;155(suppl 1):S131−S137. https://doi.org/10.1530/eje.1.02231.
10. Hembree WC, Cohen-Kettenis P, Delemarre-Van De Waal HA, et al. Endocrine treatment of transsexual persons: an endocrine society clinical practice guideline. *J Clin Endocrinol Metab.* 2009;94(9):3132−3154. https://doi.org/10.1210/jc.2009-0345.
11. Leibowitz SF, Telingator C. Assessing gender identity concerns in children and adolescents: evaluation, treatments, and outcomes. *Curr Psychiatry Rep.* 2012;14(2):111−120. https://doi.org/10.1007/s11920-012-0259-x.
12. Abel BS. Hormone treatment of children and adolescents with gender dysphoria: an ethical analysis. *Hastings Cent Rep.* 2014;44:S23−S27. https://doi.org/10.1002/hast.366.
13. NIH grant 1R01HD082554-01A1.
14. Collogan L, Fleischman A. Ethics and Research with Children: A Case-based Approach. In: Kodish E, ed. Oxford: Oxford University Press; 2005.
15. Field MJ, Behrman RE, Children I of M (US) C on CRI. Ethical Conduct of Clinical Research Involving Children; 2004. https://doi.org/10.17226/10958.
16. National Institutes of Health. The Belmont report. *Belmont Rep Ethical Princ Guidel Prot Hum Subj Res.* February 1976;1979:4−6. https://doi.org/10.1002/9780471462422.eoct093.
17. Mustanski B. Ethical and regulatory issues with conducting sexuality research with LGBT adolescents: a call to action for a scientifically informed approach. *Arch Sex Behav.* 2011;40(4):673−686. https://doi.org/10.1007/s10508-011-9745-1.

18. Holm S. *Principles of Biomedical Ethics*. 5th edn. Beauchamp TL, Childress JF. Oxford University Press; 2001:454, pound 19.95. ISBN 0-19-514332-9. *J Med Ethics*. 2002;28(5):332-NaN-332. https://doi.org/10.1136/jme.28.5.332-a.

19. de Vries ALC, McGuire JK, Steensma TD, Wagenaar ECF, Doreleijers TAH, Cohen-Kettenis PT. Young adult psychological outcome after puberty suppression and gender reassignment. *Pediatrics*. 2014;134(4):696−704. https://doi.org/10.1542/peds.2013-2958.

20. Heger S, Partsch CJ, Sippell WG. Long-term outcome after depot gonadotropin-releasing hormone agonist treatment of central precocious puberty: final height, body proportions, body composition, bone mineral density, and reproductive function. *J Clin Endocrinol Metab*. 1999; 84(12):4583−4590. http://ovidsp.ovid.com/ovidweb.cgi?T=JS&PAGE=reference&D=emed4&NEWS=N&AN=2000315277.

21. Klink D, Caris M, Heijboer A, Van Trotsenburg M, Rotteveel J. Bone mass in young adulthood following gonadotropin-releasing hormone analog treatment and cross-sex hormone treatment in adolescents with gender dysphoria. *J Clin Endocrinol Metab*. 2015;100(2): E270−E275. https://doi.org/10.1210/jc.2014-2439.

22. McDougall RJ, Gillam L, Delany C, Jayasinghe Y. Ethics of fertility preservation for prepubertal children: should clinicians offer procedures where efficacy is largely unproven? *J Med Ethics*. 2017:1−5. https://doi.org/10.1136/medethics-2016-104042.

23. Lazar L, Meyerovitch J, De Vries L, Phillip M, Lebenthal Y. Treated and untreated women with idiopathic precocious puberty: long-term follow-up and reproductive outcome between the third and fifth decades. *Clin Endocrinol (Oxf)*. 2014;80(4):570−576. https://doi.org/10.1111/cen.12319.

24. Nahata L, Tishelman AC, Caltabellotta NM, Quinn GP. Low fertility preservation utilization among transgender youth. *J Adolesc Health*. 2017;61(1):40−44. https://doi.org/10.1016/j.jadohealth.2016.12.012.

25. Dickey Lore M, Ducheny KM, Ehrbar RD. Family creation options for transgender and gender nonconforming people. *Psychol Sex Orientat Gend Divers*. 2016;3(2): 173−179. https://doi.org/10.1037/sgd0000178.

26. De Sutter P, Kira K, Verschoor A, Hotimsky A. The desire to have children and the preservation of fertility in transsexual women: a survey. *Int J Transgend*. 2002;6(3):1−12. http://www.symposion.com/ijt/ijtvo06no03_02.htm.

27. Wierckx K, Van Caenegem E, Pennings G, et al. Reproductive wish in transsexual men. *Hum Reprod*. 2012;27(2): 483−487. https://doi.org/10.1093/humrep/der406.

28. von Doussa H, Power J, Riggs D. Imagining parenthood: the possibilities and experiences of parenthood among transgender people. *Cult Health Sex*. 2015;17(9):1119−1131. https://doi.org/10.1080/13691058.2015.1042919.

29. Katz AL, Webb SA. Informed consent in decision-making in pediatric practice. *Pediatrics*. 2016;138(2):e20161485. https://doi.org/10.1542/peds.2016-1485.

30. Steensma TD, McGuire JK, Kreukels BPC, Beekman AJ, Cohen-Kettenis PT. Factors associated with desistence and persistence of childhood gender dysphoria: a quantitative follow-up study. *J Am Acad Child Adolesc Psychiatry*. 2013; 52(6):582−590. https://doi.org/10.1016/j.jaac.2013.03.016.

31. Kyrios M, Moulding R, Doron G, Bhar SS, Nedeljkovic M, Mikulincer M, eds. *The Self in Understanding and Treating Psychological Disorders*. Cambridge: Cambridge University Press; 2016. https://doi.org/10.1017/CBO9781139941297.

CHAPTER 12

Emerging Developments in Pubertal Suppression for Gender Incongruent/Gender Dysphoric Youth

MAJA MARINKOVIC, MD • JEREMI CARSWELL, MD • STEPHANIE A. ROBERTS, MD

TRIPTORELIN, A NEW GONADOTROPIN-RELEASING HORMONE AGONIST

The use of gonadotropin-releasing hormone (GnRH) agonists for suppressing puberty for gender dysphoric/gender-incongruent youth is an established part of the treatment protocols.[1,2] In addition to previously approved GnRH agonists, since late 2017, clinicians have one more agonist available for suppression of sex hormones.

Triptorelin, a synthetic decapeptide analog of GnRH, has been available in Europe since 1986 and more recently, as of 2017, has been approved for use in the United States. Triptorelin, as monthly and every 3-monthly preparations, has been used for treatment of central precocious puberty (CPP),[3,4] endometriosis,[5] and neoplasms of the breast and prostate. Additionally, triptorelin is the primary GnRH agonist used for pubertal suppression in youth with gender dysphoria in many European countries.[6,7]

Triptorelin, marketed in the United States as Triptodur (22.5 mg per dose), is a long-acting analog intramuscular injection. Its benefit over other forms of injected GnRH agonist is that it has a prolonged duration of action, requiring administration only every 24 weeks.[8] Its safety and efficacy for treatment of children with CPP was established in an international trial.[9] The use of Triptodur (or any other GnRH agonist) for pubertal suppression in gender dysphoric youth is not approved by the Food and Drug Administration (FDA), and currently, there are no data available on its use in this specific population. Following the first dose, as it was demonstrated with other GnRH agonists, a phase of pubertal stimulation can be observed before pubertal suppression is achieved and patients should be counseled accordingly.[8] Intramuscular application has been associated with pain at the injection site in about

half of the patients, together with occasional pruritus, erythema, and swelling. In addition, some patients experienced emotional lability, irritability, anger, and aggression while on treatment. This may be particularly relevant for patients with gender dysphoria who have coexisting depression and anxiety; however, mood symptoms may theoretically improve if gender dysphoria improves on GnRH agonist therapy. Continued counseling/therapy and close follow-up is advised during the treatment. There have been reports of hypertension associated with the use of triptorelin in CPP and regular monitoring is advised.[10,11] Poor bone health related to prolonged use of this and other GnRH agonists in gender dysphoric youth is another concern. Limited reports indicate a decrease in bone mineral density, particularly in European transwomen treated with triptorelin 3.75 mg every 4 weeks until gonadectomy.[12] Larger long-term studies are needed to further investigate efficacy, safety, and possible side effects of triptorelin, especially in gender dysphoric youth.

PROLONGED USE OF HISTRELIN ACETATE IMPLANT IN TRANSGENDER YOUTH

Histrelin acetate implant (Supprelin® LA, 50 mg) has been approved for treatment of CPP in the United States since 2007 and has been shown to be an effective, potent pubertal suppressor. It is approved for a 1-year duration; however, it has been demonstrated in clinical practice that the implant can remain effective for longer periods (e.g., 2–3 years) in some patients with CPP[13] and prostate cancer.[14,15] Published data on its extended use in gender-incongruent population are lacking.

There are several potential benefits from keeping the implant in place beyond 1 year: reduced frequency of anesthesia (general, local), fewer surgical interventions required, and dramatic decrease in overall cost of treatment. Additionally, reduction of replacement frequency could significantly improve some transgender-health relatedaccess to adequate care, as this implant is only covered by insurance in a limited number of states.[16] Potential risks of prolonged implantation include resumption of some transgender-health relatedpuberty (and potentially irreversible physical effects), as well as an increased level of difficulty in its removal, occasionally leading to retained pieces of an embedded device. An increased frequency of clinical exams and, potentially, blood tests are needed to closely monitor success of pubertal suppression. The risks and benefits of annual replacement versus extended use should be carefully discussed with each patient and their family.

GONADOTROPIN-RELEASING HORMONE AGONIST USE IN NONBINARY YOUTH

Increasingly, youth are identifying outside of an affirmed gender as solely male or female, and on the gender spectrum as nonbinary.[17] Currently guidelines do not provide guidance on this population of youth; however, clinical care is driven by helping a youth achieve their goals within the confines of available medical therapies.

Within the nonbinary spectrum, including youth who may identify as agender, the use of GnRH analogs to eliminate effects of unwanted sex steroids may be considered as a treatment option not only as a "pause" to allow a child more time to explore gender but also for individuals who may desire to live in an agonadal state. Prolonged exposure in an agonadal state due to GnRH agonist without concomitant use of either estrogen or testosterone is not recommended and should be exercised with extreme caution given the lack of available safety data and risk of causing harm, including psychosocial impact and potential negative impact on long-term bone mineral density and future fracture risk.

GONADOTROPIN-RELEASING HORMONE AND GONADOTROPIN ANTAGONISTS

Inhibition of the GnRH receptor (as opposed to stimulation as occurs with GnRH agonists) is also an effective means to prevent activation of the hypothalamic–pituitary–gonadal (HPG) axis. GnRH antagonists have similar side effects to GnRH agonists; however, they offer the advantage of a rapid decline in gonadal steroid production and avoidance of the surge in luteinizing hormone and follicle stimulating hormone, and therefore, downstream gonadal steroid production.[18] There are several forms of GnRH receptor antagonist commercially available in the United States, primarily limited to use in prostate cancer, infertility treatment, and endometriosis. There is no published experience of the use of GnRH antagonists in CPP or transgender care, and they are not FDA approved for youth. Its use has been limited by cost, availability, and mode of administration which is a moderate-volume monthly subcutaneous or intramuscular injection. An orally active form is currently in clinical trial for moderate-to-severe endometriosis.[20]

Gonadotropin Antagonists

Upon activation, the GnRH receptor acts to stimulate the release of luteinizing hormone receptor and follicle-stimulating hormone. Thus, antagonists of the gonadotropin (luteinizing hormone and follicle-stimulating hormone) receptors are also potential therapeutic targets but are in the early stages of development.[21]

KISSPEPTIN AND NEUROKININ B ANTAGONISTS

Other hormones acting upstream above the level of GnRH are also potential therapeutic targets to achieve pubertal blockade. Kisspeptin, one of GnRH's most potent activators, is produced in the hypothalamus and is also an important player in pubertal onset.[22] Children with loss-of-function or inactivating mutations in kisspeptin or its receptor exhibit delayed puberty.[23] Thus, inhibiting kisspeptin or the kisspeptin receptor are also potential therapeutic targets.[19]

Kisspeptin and kisspeptin receptor antagonists are available in a research setting, mainly used in rodent experiments, and could foreseeably be available to treat human disease in the near future.[24] Importantly, the inhibition of gonadotropin secretion and downstream gonadal effects may not be as complete as GnRH agonists or antagonists, as there appears to be some kisspeptin-independent secretion of GnRH. Kisspeptin antagonists appear to reduce pulsatility of luteinizing hormone, thereby leading to diminished ovulation, but does not appear to inhibit basal luteinizing hormone secretion which could have therapeutic implications of lowering sex steroids while avoiding adverse effects of complete gonadal suppression.[25]

Neurokinin B is a positive regulator of GnRH and is coexpressed by the same neurons in the hypothalamus that secrete kisspeptin. Inhibition of neurokinin B or its receptor, neurokinin-3 receptor, is another potential strategy for pubertal suppression. In parallel to kisspeptin, loss-of-function mutations in the genes encoding neurokinin B or its receptor lead to delayed puberty, thus inhibition of these targets could lead to suppression of the gonadal steroid production.[26] The use of a neurokinin-3 receptor antagonist has been shown to decrease sex hormones in healthy men and women.[27] Neurokinin-3 receptor antagonists are currently in clinical trials for use in perimenopausal women experiencing hot flashes.[28]

OXANDROLONE AS AN ALTERNATIVE GENDER-AFFIRMING MASCULINIZING HORMONE

As a non-aromatizable synthetic analog of the potent androgen 5-α dihydrotestosterone, oxandrolone is approved by the FDA to "offset protein catabolism associated with prolonged administration of corticosteroids, and [to provide] relief of the bone pain frequently accompanying osteoporosis."[29] Despite these relatively narrow indications, oxandrolone has gained favor in pediatrics, particularly in two distinct populations: burn victims for prevention of catabolism and girls with Turner syndrome for height gain. Literature from both populations has informed the consideration of this agent in the transmasculine population for the purpose of increasing height.[30,31]

The structure of this synthetic molecule is not susceptible to the aromatase enzyme, whose role is to catalyze androgens to estrogens. It therefore maintains its androgenic effects, but, importantly, will not contribute the estrogenic effect of epiphyseal fusion at the growth plates. In turn, this theoretically preserves the open growth plates and allows for prolonged growth. The use of oxandrolone found favor early on in the Turner syndrome population as untreated girls will have a final height that is about 20 cm below expected.[32-35] Early studies noted virilization (e.g., increased clitoral size and increased body hair) as a side effect, but the use of a low dose of oxandrolone (0.03 mg/kg per day) resulted in an increased height gain without much risk for masculinization.[36,37] Recently published guidelines for Turner syndrome recommend the use of this agent, in conjunction with growth hormone, for optimization of height gain in the following situations: if predicted height is very short and/or in the case of delayed diagnosis and growth hormone initiation.[38]

Oxandrolone use in transmasculine youth has not been studied to our knowledge, but it has gained traction for use in this population. The group of patients who may benefit the most are young peripubertal transmales whose growth has not completed and who are concomitantly on GnRH agonists. Allowing longer time for growth (the effect of pubertal suppression in these youth) in addition to mild anabolic and growth-promoting effects of oxandrolone, in theory, could have a positive impact on the final height. The effects of oxandrolone related to virilization (increase in muscle mass, body hairs, and clitoral size) would be advantageous in this population. It is important to note that when oxandrolone is used in cisgender boys with constitutional delay of growth and puberty to promote height, the results are mixed.[39-44]

As mentioned, side effects are primarily related to virilization, although this may be a dose-dependent phenomenon and likely would be a desired effect in transmales.[37,45,46] Virilization includes acne, voice deepening, and clitoromegaly, as well as decreased high-density lipoprotein levels. Additional risks of oxandrolone use include idiosyncratic drug-induced liver injury, cholestatic hepatitis, and jaundice, as well as longer term risk for peliosis hepatis which can lead to hepatic dysfunction ranging from mild liver damage to liver failure.[29]

In sum, while the use of oxandrolone presents a potential way to maximize height potential and provide mild masculinizing effects prior to starting testosterone, clinical studies looking into its effect and safety should be conducted before it can be recommended for routine use.

LOW-DOSE ESTROGEN AND TESTOSTERONE

The role of low-dose estrogen or testosterone has been suggested in two populations; the first is for promotion of bone health in those with low bone mineral density due to prolonged sex steroid deprivation (e.g., those who had GnRH agonist treatment initiated at a very young age) and those who desire only modest effect of sex hormones.

The use of very-low-dose transdermal estradiol has been studied in a hypogonadal population and has been found to mimic the physiologic levels of estrogen seen in cis-girls with intact HPGs. One early study noted breast development within 3 months of estradiol use in 2/3 of girls.[47] This finding was replicated in another study with doses of transdermal estradiol ranging from 3.1 to 6.2 μg/24 h placed only overnight.[48] There are no discrete data in these studies on bone density, although it seems reasonable to assume that this small amount of estrogen would have a positive effect on the bone; the magnitude and later impact are unknown. Current guidelines do not, however, recommend its routine use.[38]

Similarly, the use of low-dose testosterone has not been studied for the purposes of either improving bone density or for partial masculinization for nonbinary individuals with gender dysphoria. A slow increase of testosterone starting at 25 mg intramuscularly once monthly has been proposed for hypogonadal cisgender boys, but the effects of low doses on bone mineral density have not been studied.[49]

ANTIANDROGENS AND ANDROGEN RECEPTOR INHIBITORS

Spironolactone, a potassium-sparing diuretic with mild antiandrogen properties, has been a well-established component of feminizing treatment protocols,[1,2] particularly when more potent antiandrogens are not available. Spironolactone is a competitive antagonist of aldosterone at the mineralocorticoid receptor. It also interferes with testosterone biosynthesis by reducing 17-hydroxylase activity, as well as inhibiting binding of dihydrotestosterone, the more active form of testosterone.[51] As opposed to the antiandrogens below, the levels of measured testosterone would be expected to decrease. It is inexpensive, relatively safe, and, in combination with estrogen, effective in androgen suppression for most patients. This makes spironolactone an attractive alternative to GnRH agonist; however, increased urination, risk of hypotension, and hyperkalemia, as well as incomplete androgen suppression in some cases necessitates use of alternate treatments.

ANTIANDROGENS

Agents that interfere either with the production or action of testosterone are potential targets for intervention for the transfeminine identified patient. As a class, the antiandrogens (bicalutamide, flutamide, and nilutamide) bind directly to the androgen receptor, thereby inhibiting its availability and increasing the receptors' degradation.[50] The primary indication is for metastatic prostate cancer, although it has been used in the transfeminine population.[52] These three agents differ primarily by pharmacokinetics, bicalutamide having the longest duration of action. While on the medication, testosterone levels are expected to rise dramatically but do not have an effect. Gynecomastia is a recognized side effect and could be desired in the transfeminine population. There are cases of fulminant

hepatitis described, and it is recommended that transaminase levels are checked prior to initiation and then at 4-month intervals.[53] The use of antiandrogens has not been rigorously studied in the gender nonconforming population, but its use is recommended for consideration in some transgender-health related publications.[54–56]

CONCLUSION

There are many agents that have been used in other areas of medicine that may be promising as potential therapies for transgender and gender-incongruent youth. Until safety can be demonstrated, we recommend limiting their use until such studies have been performed or more traditional options have been tried.

REFERENCES

1. Hembree WC, Cohen-Kettenis PT, Gooren L, et al. *J Clin Endocrinol Metab.* 2017;102(11):3869–3903.
2. Coleman E, Bockting W, Botzer M, et al. WPATH-"Standards of care" (SOC) version 7. *Int J Transgend.* 2011;13:165–232.
3. Boucekkine C, Blumberg-Tick J, Roger M, Thomas F, Chaussain JL. Treatment of central precocious puberty with sustained-release triptorelin. *Arch Pediatr.* 1994;1(12):1127–1137.
4. Carel JC, Blumberg J, Seymour C, Adamsbaum C, Lahlou N. Triptorelin 3-month CPP Study Group. Three-month sustained-release triptorelin (11.25 mg) in the treatment of central precocious puberty. *Eur J Endocrinol.* 2006;154(1):119–124.
5. Bergqvist A, Bergh T, Hogström L, Mattsson S, Nordenskjöld F, Rasmussen C. Effects of triptorelin versus placebo on the symptoms of endometriosis. *Fertil Steril.* 1998;69(4):702–708.
6. Cohen-Kettenis PT, Klink D. Adolescents with gender dysphoria. *Best Pract Res Clin Endocrinol Metab.* 2015;29(3):485–495.
7. Schagen SE, Cohen-Kettenis PT, Delemarre-van de Waal HA, Hannema SE. Efficacy and safety of gonadotropin-releasing hormone agonist treatment to suppress puberty in gender dysphoric adolescents. *J Sex Med.* 2016;13(7):1125–1132.
8. *Triptodur [package insert].* Atlanta, GA: Arbor Pharmaceuticals, LLC.
9. Klein K, Yang J, Aisenberg J, et al. Efficacy and safety of triptorelin 6-month formulation in patients with central precocious puberty. *J Pediatr Endocrinol Metab.* 2016;29(11):1241–1248.
10. Calcaterra V, Mannarino S, Corana G, et al. Hypertension during therapy with triptorelin in a girl with precocious puberty. *Indian J Pediatr.* 2013;80(10):884–885.

11. Siomou E, Kosmeri C, Pavlou M, Vlahos AP, Argyropoulou MI, Siamopoulou A. Arterial hypertension during treatment with triptorelin in a child with Williams-Beuren syndrome. *Pediatr Nephrol.* 2014;29(9): 1633–1636.

12. Klink D, Caris M, Heijboer A, van Trotsenburg M, Rotteveel J. Bone mass in young adulthood following gonadotropin-releasing hormone analog treatment and cross-sex hormone treatment in adolescents with gender dysphoria. *J Clin Endocrinol Metab.* 2015;100(2): E270–E275.

13. Lewis KA, Goldyn AK, West KW, Eugster EA. A single Histrelin implant is effective for 2 years for treatment of central precocious puberty. *J Pediatr.* 2013;163(4): 1214–1216.

14. Chertin B, Spitz IM, Lindenberg T, et al. An implant releasing the gonadotropin hormone-releasing hormone agonist histrelin maintains medical castration for up to 30 months in metastatic prostate cancer. *J Urol.* 2000; 163(3):838–844.

15. Schlegel PN, Kuzma P, Frick J, et al. Effective long-term androgen suppression in men with prostate cancer using a hydrogel implant with the GnRH agonist histrelin. *Urology.* 2001;58(4):578–582.

16. Nahata L, Quinn GP, Caltabellotta NM, Tishelman AC. Mental health concerns and insurance denials among transgender adolescents. *LGBT Health.* 2017;4(3): 188–193.

17. Eckstrand KL, Ng H, Potter J. Affirmative and responsible health care for people with nonconforming gender identities and expressions. *AMA J Ethic.* 2016;18: 1107–1118.

18. Ron-El R, Raziel A, Schachter M, Strassburger D, Kasterstein E, Friedler S. Induction of ovulation after GnRH antagonists. *Hum Reprod Update.* 2000;6(4): 318–321.

19. Newton CL, Anderson RC, Millar RP. Therapeutic neuroendocrine agonist and antagonist analogs of hypothalamic neuropeptides as modulators of the hypothalamic-pituitary-gonadal axis. *Endocr Dev.* 2016;30:106–129. https://doi.org/10.1159/000439337.

20. Taylor HS, Giudice LC, Lessey BA, et al. Treatment of endometriosis-associated pain with elagolix, an oral GnRH antagonist. *N Engl J Med.* 2017;377:28–40.

21. Guo T. Small molecule agonists and antagonists for the LH and FSH receptors. *Expert Opin Ther Pat.* 2005;15: 1555–1564.

22. Dungan HM, Clifton DK, Steiner RA. Minireview: kisspeptin neurons as central processors in the regulation of gonadotropin-releasing hormone secretion. *Endocrinology.* 2006;147:1154–1158.

23. Bianco SDC, Kaiser UB. The genetic and molecular basis of idiopathic hypogonadotropic hypogonadism. *Nat Rev Endocrinol.* 2009;5:569–576.

24. Roseweir AK, Millar RP. Kisspeptin antagonists. *Adv Exp Med Biol.* 2013;784:159–186.

25. Pineda R, Garcia-Galiano D, Roseweir A, et al. Critical roles of kisspeptin in female puberty and preovulatory gonadotropin surges as revealed by a novel antagonist. *J Clin Endocrinol Metab.* 2009;94:5181.

26. Gianetti E, Tusset C, Noel SD, et al. TAC3/TACR3Mutations reveal preferential activation of gonadotropin-releasing hormone release by neurokinin B in neonatal life followed by reversal in adulthood. *J Clin Endocrinol Metab.* 2010;95:2857–2867.

27. Fraser GL, Ramael S, Hoveyda HR, Gheyle L, Combalbert J. The NK3 receptor antagonist ESN364 suppresses sex hormones in men and women. *J Clin Endocrinol Metab.* 2016;101:417–426.

28. Skorupskaite K, George JT, Veldhuis JD, Millar RP, Anderson RA. Neurokinin 3 receptor antagonism reveals roles for neurokinin B in the regulation of gonadotropin secretion and hot flashes in postmenopausal women. *Neuroendocrinology.* 2017;106.

29. *Product Information: Oxandrolone Oral Tablets, Oxandrolone Oral Tablets.* Maple Grove, MN: Upsher-Smith Laboratories Inc. (per DailyMed); 2015.

30. Cohen-Kettenis PT, Delemarre-van de Waal HA, Gooren LJG. The treatment of adolescent transsexuals: changing insights. *J Sex Med.* 2008;5(8):1892–1897. https://doi.org/10.1111/j.1743-6109.2008.00870.x.

31. Delemarre-van de Waal HA, Cohen-Kettenis PT. Clinical management of gender identity disorder in adolescents: a protocol on psychological and paediatric endocrinology aspects. *Eur J Endocrinol.* 2006;155(suppl 1):S131–S137. https://doi.org/10.1530/eje.1.02231.

32. Lyon AJ, Preece MA, Grant DB. Growth curve for girls with Turner syndrome. *Arch Dis Child.* 1985;60(10):932–935. http://www.ncbi.nlm.nih.gov/pubmed/4062345.

33. Saari A, Sankilampi U, Dunkel L. Multiethnic WHO growth charts may not be optimal in the screening of disorders affecting height: Turner syndrome as a model. *JAMA Pediatr.* 2013;167(2):194. https://doi.org/10.1001/jamapediatrics.2013.436.

34. Bertapelli F, Barros-Filho Ade A, Antonio MÂ, Barbeta CJ, de Lemos-Marini SH, Guerra-Junior G. Growth curves for girls with Turner syndrome. *Biomed Res Int.* 2014;2014: 687978. https://doi.org/10.1155/2014/687978.

35. Yang S. Diagnostic and therapeutic considerations in Turner syndrome. *Ann Pediatr Endocrinol Metab.* 2017;22(4): 226–230. https://doi.org/10.6065/apem.2017.22.4.226.

36. Freriks K, Sas TCJ, Traas MAF, et al. Long-term effects of previous oxandrolone treatment in adult women with Turner syndrome. *Eur J Endocrinol.* 2012;168(1):91–99. https://doi.org/10.1530/EJE-12-0404.

37. Sas TCJ, Gault EJ, Zeger Bardsley M, et al. Safety and efficacy of oxandrolone in growth hormone-treated girls with Turner syndrome: evidence from recent studies and recommendations for use. *Horm Res Paediatr.* 2014; 81(5):289–297. https://doi.org/10.1159/000358195.

38. Gravholt CH, Andersen NH, Conway GS, et al. Clinical practice guidelines for the care of girls and women with Turner syndrome: proceedings from the 2016 Cincinnati International Turner Syndrome Meeting. *Eur J Endocrinol.* 2017;177(3):G1–G70. https://doi.org/10.1530/EJE-17-0430.

39. Salehpour S, Alipour P, Razzaghy-Azar M, et al. A double-blind, placebo-controlled comparison of letrozole to oxandrolone effects upon growth and puberty of children with constitutional delay of puberty and idiopathic short stature. *Horm Res Paediatr.* 2010;74(6):428–435. https://doi.org/10.1159/000315482.

40. Sheanon NM, Backeljauw PF. Effect of oxandrolone therapy on adult height in Turner syndrome patients treated with growth hormone: a meta-analysis. *Int J Pediatr Endocrinol.* 2015;2015(1):18. https://doi.org/10.1186/s13633-015-0013-3.

41. Albanese A, Kewley GD, Long A, Pearl KN, Robins DG, Stanhope R. Oral treatment for constitutional delay of growth and puberty in boys: a randomized trial of an anabolic steroid or testosterone undecanoate. *Arch Dis Child.* 1994;71:315–317.

42. Schroor EJ, van Weissenbruch MM, Knibbe P, Delemarre-van de Waal HA. The effect of prolonged administration of an anabolic steroid (oxandrolone) on growth in boys with constitutionally delayed growth. *Eur J Pediatr.* 1995;154(12):953–957.

43. Wilson DM, McCauley E, Brown DR, Dudley R. Oxandrolone therapy in constitutionally delayed growth and puberty. Bio-technology general corporation cooperative study group. *Pediatrics.* 1995;96(6):1095–1100.

44. Stanhope R, Buchanan CR, Fenn GC, Preece MA. Double blind placebo controlled trial of low dose oxandrolone in the treatment of boys with constitutional delay of growth and puberty. *Arch Dis Child.* 1988;63(5):501–505.

45. Menke LA, Sas TCJ, de Muinck Keizer-Schrama SMPF, et al. Efficacy and safety of oxandrolone in growth hormone-treated girls with Turner syndrome. *J Clin Endocrinol Metab.* 2010;95(3):1151–1160. https://doi.org/10.1210/jc.2009-1821.

46. Zeger MPD, Shah K, Kowal K, Cutler GB, Kushner H, Ross JL. Prospective study confirms oxandrolone-associated improvement in height in growth hormone-treated adolescent girls with Turner syndrome. *Horm Res Paediatr.* 2011;75(1):38–46. https://doi.org/10.1159/000317529.

47. Illig R, DeCampo C, Lang-Muritano MR, et al. A physiological mode of puberty induction in hypogonadal girls by low dose transdermal 17 beta-oestradiol. *Eur J Pediatr.* 1990;150(2):86–91. http://www.ncbi.nlm.nih.gov/pubmed/2126236.

48. Ankarberg-Lindgren C, Elfving M, Wikland KA, Norjavaara E. Nocturnal application of transdermal estradiol patches produces levels of estradiol that mimic those seen at the onset of spontaneous puberty in girls. *J Clin Endocrinol Metab.* 2001;86(7):3039–3044. https://doi.org/10.1210/jcem.86.7.7667.

49. Sato N, Hasegawa T, Hasegawa Y, et al. Treatment situation of male hypogonadotropic hypogonadism in pediatrics and proposal of testosterone and gonadotropins replacement therapy protocols. *Clin Pediatr Endocrinol.* 2015;24(2):37–49. https://doi.org/10.1297/cpe.24.37.

50. Drug Result Page—MICROMEDEX® Bicalutamide. http://www.micromedexsolutions.com/micromedex2/librarian/CS/DB6536/ND_PR/evidencexpert/ND_P/evidencexpert/DUPLICATIONSHIELDSYNC/4D7C97/ND_PG/evidencexpert/ND_B/evidencexpert/ND_AppProduct/evidencexpert/ND_T/evidencexpert/PFActionId/evidencexpert.DoIntegra.

51. Loriaux DL, Menard R, Taylor A, et al. Spironolactone and endocrine dysfunction. *Ann Intern Med.* 1976;85:630–636.

52. Neyman A, Fuqua JS, Eugster EA. 10th individual abstracts for international meeting of pediatric endocrinology: free communication and poster sessions, abstracts. *Horm Res Paediatr.* 2017;88(suppl 1):1–628. https://doi.org/10.1159/000481424.

53. Product Information: Bicalutamide Oral Tablets, Bicalutamide Oral Tablets. Northstar Rx LLC, Memphis, TN, 2011.

54. Gooren LJ. Care of transsexual persons. *N Engl J Med.* 2011;364(13):1251–1257. https://doi.org/10.1056/NEJMcp1008161.

55. Wierckx K, Gooren L, T'Sjoen G. Clinical review: breast development in trans women receiving cross-sex hormones. *J Sex Med.* 2014;11(5):1240–1247. https://doi.org/10.1111/jsm.12487.

56. Deutsch M. *Guidelines for the Primary and Gender Affirming Care of Transgender and Gender Nonconforming People: Overview of Feminizing Hormone Therapy;* 2016. http://transhealth.ucsf.edu/trans?page=guidelines-feminizing-therapy.

Index

Note: Page numbers followed by "f" indicate figures, "t" indicate tables.

Printed in the United States
By Bookmasters